In NATURE *We* TRUST

A Raw Food Manifesto for Energy, Healing & Longevity

Axay Shah

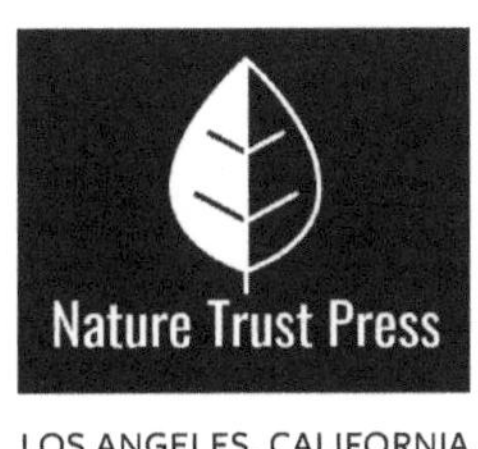

LOS ANGELES, CALIFORNIA

Published by Nature Trust Press
An imprint of Nature Press LLC
Los Angeles, California
NatureTrustPress.com

IN NATURE WE TRUST® is a registered trademark of Akshay Shah
U.S. Trademark Registration No. 8116488
Registered January 27, 2026

ISBN 979–8-9940378–0-5 (Paperback)
ISBN 979–8-9940378–1-2 (Hardcover)
ISBN 979–8-9940378–2-9 (Ebook)

Library of Congress Control Number: 2026907840

DISCLAIMER: The information contained in this book is based on the author's personal experience and research. It is not intended as a substitute for professional medical advice. Readers should consult their healthcare providers before making any dietary changes.

Cover and interior design by Happenstance Type-O-Rama

Printed in the United States of America
First Edition, 2026

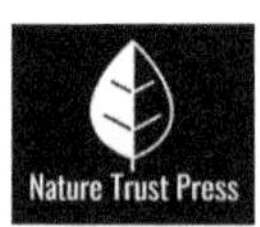

NatureTrustPress.com
RawFoodiest.com
InNatureWeTrust.net

ONE WITH NATURE

To Mother Nature

This manifesto exists because of you.

Every insight in these pages about energy, about healing, about the true nature of health comes from understanding how you designed us. How, over millions of years of evolution, you created bodies that thrive on whole plant foods as you provide them. How you engineered mitochondria to extract perfect energy from nature's abundance. How you built within us the wisdom to heal ourselves when we finally stop fighting you and start listening.

This book is not my creation. It is a reflection of your creation. I am simply translating what you have been trying to tell us all along—that you know how to sustain life. That your design works. That when we align with you instead of against you, health is the natural result.

For over sixteen years of my own journey, and over twenty-one years of documented transformation in my body and mind, I have experienced this truth: *In Nature We Trust* is not philosophy or marketing. It is an observable reality. It is what happens when humans stop trying to outsmart you and instead cooperate with you.

Every person who reverses disease through this protocol is not fighting against nature. They are finally surrendering to it. They are finally saying yes to what you have been offering all along.

This manifesto is dedicated to you, Mother Nature. Not as distant reverence, but as practical gratitude. Thank you for designing a body that can heal. Thank you for providing foods that nourish perfectly. Thank you for the intelligence you built into every cell, every mitochondrion, every system waiting patiently for us to finally listen.

And to everyone who reads this manifesto: Mother Nature did not make a mistake when she made you. Your body and mind are not broken. Your body is waiting for you to provide what it actually needs. When you do, you will experience what I have experienced, what thousands have experienced: the profound healing that comes from finally trusting the design that created you.

In Nature We Trust.

Life is Energy and Energy is Life.

With deepest reverence and gratitude,
AXAY SHAH

CONTENTS

SECTION 1: **PHILOSOPHICAL FOUNDATION**
Understanding Energy as the Root of All Health

SECTION 2: **ENERGY RESTORATION PROTOCOL**
Practical Implementation of the Energy Restoration Framework

SECTION 3: MY TRANSFORMATION JOURNEY
From Decision Through Achievement to Thriving—
The Proof of What Energy Restoration Creates in Real Life

SECTION 4: YOUR TRANSFORMATION AND INTEGRATION
Applying the Protocol to Your Life, Your Circumstances, Your Future

FOREWORD

In *In Nature We Trust*, readers are invited on an enlightening journey through the profound relationship between nature, health, and wellness. This book stands out as a comprehensive guide, meticulously detailing the causes of diseases and presenting practical strategies to reverse them. Its systematic approach caters to individuals from all walks of life and across all age groups, making it an invaluable resource for anyone seeking personal transformation.

The author's commitment to exploring various nutritional aspects, particularly the benefits of a raw food diet, offers deep insight into how our dietary choices can shape our health. This book serves as a beacon of knowledge, empowering readers to embrace nature's offerings and make informed decisions that promote healing and vitality.

In Nature We Trust is more than just a guide; it is a vital companion for those ready to take charge of their health and embark on a path of renewal. Whether you are just beginning your journey towards better health or looking to deepen your understanding of plant-based lifestyles, this book is a true gem in the world of nutrition. It is a testament to the power of nature and the endless possibilities it holds for our well-being.

May this book inspire and motivate you to trust in nature, unlock your potential, and embrace a healthier, more vibrant life.

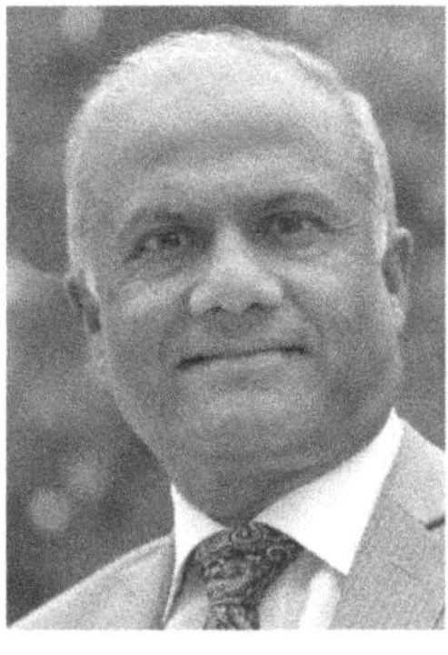

—DR. SHRENIK SHAH, MD

INTRODUCTION

Why I Wrote This Manifesto

My name is Axay Shah. At the time of writing this, I'm sixty-six years young. I've completed seven marathons and I'm training for my eighth. I have the energy and physical capacity of someone in their forties. My blood pressure is optimal. My blood glucose is perfect. My cognitive function is sharp. My mood is stable. I sleep deeply. I have no medications. I have no chronic disease.

This is not because I'm genetically blessed. This is not because I'm special. This is because for the past sixteen plus years, I have been living an energy-aligned life. And over the past twenty-one plus years, I have meticulously documented what happens to the human body when it receives what it actually needs: plant-based raw foods, abundant movement, and alignment with nature.

The results have been extraordinary. Not just for me, but for thousands of people who have implemented what I'm about to share with you in this manifesto.

When I started this journey on December 6, 2009, I made a decision that changed everything: I committed to eating only foods made by Mother Nature, nothing made by industry. No processed foods. No refined carbohydrates. No extracted oils. No animal products. Just plant-based raw foods, as close to nature as possible.

I didn't know I was starting a medical experiment. I just knew I wanted to feel better.

What happened over the next sixteen years astonished me. My health didn't just improve. It transformed. Completely. My body reversed decades of dysfunction. My mind became clear. My energy became abundant. And I began to understand something profound: I hadn't been sick. I had been energy starved. My cells were drowning in inflammatory toxins while being deprived of the nutrients they actually needed.

When I fixed that, when I provided my body what it actually needed, everything changed.

Why Now? Why This Manifesto?

Over the past several years, I've been sharing this journey with people. Thousands of them. Through my Raw Foodiest community. Through conversations. Through the evidence of my medical data, my athletic performance at sixty-six, my lived experience.

And I started hearing the same questions over and over: "How do I start?" "Will this really work for me?" "What about my [disease, condition, circumstance]?" "How do I do this long term?" "Why does this work?"

The answers to these questions deserve to be comprehensive, detailed, evidence-based, and real.

This manifesto is my answer.

What emerged is a complete framework—a way to understand why chronic disease happens, how to reverse it, how to prevent it, and how to maintain optimal health for decades.

This framework isn't theoretical. It's practical. It's based on real transformation in real people living real lives with real obstacles and circumstances.

Who This Is For

This manifesto is for you if:

You have a chronic disease and you want to know if it can be reversed. (It can. I'll show you how.)

You're seeing warning signs of elevated blood pressure, pre-diabetes, weight gain, fatigue, or anxiety and you want to prevent the disease before it fully develops. (You can. I'll show you how.)

You're "fine" but you know something is off. You don't have the energy you used to, you're not sleeping well, you're experiencing brain fog, your mood isn't stable. (You can fix this. I'll show you how.)

You care about your family's health and you want to know how to raise children with optimal health as their baseline, or how to help aging parents reverse disease. (Both are possible. I'll show you how.)

You're tired of being told that your health is just bad luck or genetics and you want to understand that you have far more power over your health than you've been led to believe. (You do. I'll prove it to you.)

You want to understand why chronic disease is an epidemic and what the real solution is, not the symptom-management approach that dominates modern medicine. (I'll explain it clearly.)

This manifesto is for anyone willing to consider that the food they eat might be creating disease, and that different food might create health.

What You'll Experience

When you read this manifesto, here's what will happen:

You'll understand the fundamental framework that all chronic disease stems from energy system dysfunction. This single insight changes everything. It connects cardiovascular disease, obesity, diabetes, mental health conditions, cognitive decline, all of it into one unified system. You'll stop seeing disease as random and start seeing it as information.

You'll get a complete, practical protocol for restoring energy system function. Not theoretical. Practical. Step by step. Week by week. You'll know exactly what to eat, why you're eating it, what to expect as your body heals, and how to navigate obstacles.

You'll see disease reversal in real people, cardiovascular disease reversed, weight normalized, depression lifted, cognitive function restored, with medical markers tracked throughout. You'll see the timeline of healing. You'll see what's actually possible.

You'll understand disease prevention, not just as theory but also as practical reality. You'll see how one protocol prevents all diseases simultaneously because all diseases share the same root cause.

You'll get guidance for your specific circumstances, whether you're pregnant, an athlete, elderly, on a limited budget, dealing with food allergies, struggling with mental illness, or facing any other special circumstance. This isn't one-size-fits-all. It's adaptable to your life.

You'll understand how to maintain these changes for decades. Not just reverse disease for a few months, then return to previous patterns. But sustain optimal health indefinitely. You'll understand the role of movement, the importance of sustainability, and how to build a life where health is simply how you live.

You'll understand something deeper: you have power, more power over your health than you've been led to believe. That your health is not random. That you are not a victim of your genes or your circumstances. That you can choose differently, and that choice matters profoundly.

How to Use This Manifesto

You can read this from cover to cover. It's designed to build from philosophy to practical implementation to real-world transformation. Or you can jump to what you need:

- If you want to understand the why, start with Section 1 (Philosophical Foundation)

- If you want to understand the how, go straight to Section 2 (Energy Restoration Protocol)
- If you want to see it working in real people, read Section 3 (My Transformation Journey)
- If you want guidance for your specific circumstances, find your situation in Section 4 (Your Transformation and Integration)

You can read it once for understanding or reference it repeatedly as you implement.

Whatever your approach, engage with it actively. Take notes. Mark passages that resonate. Ask yourself: "How does this apply to my life?"

My Promise to You

I want to be clear about something: I'm not a medical doctor. I'm not a registered dietitian. I'm a man who has spent sixteen plus years living this protocol, twenty-one plus years documenting my transformation, and several years working with thousands of people as they've implemented it.

What I am is a messenger. I'm telling you what I know to be true because I've lived it, I've seen it repeated across thousands of people, and I believe you deserve to know it.

Everything in this manifesto is grounded in:

- Real medical data (my own twenty-one plus years of documented transformation)
- Scientific understanding (the mechanisms of energy system dysfunction and restoration)
- Practical guidance (not theory, but what actually works)

My promise is that this manifesto will give you a complete framework for understanding your health, the power to transform it, and the practical guidance to do so.

A Personal Note

I've spent most of my professional career in the diamonds, jewelry, and home improvement industries. It's a good living. I've been successful. But my real passion, my true calling has always been health and wellness.

Over the past several years, that passion has evolved into Raw Foodiest, a mission to share what I've learned, to support others in reclaiming their health, to demonstrate that disease is not inevitable, and to help create a future where chronic disease becomes rare rather than common.

This manifesto is part of that mission.

I'm not trying to convince you that you need to do this. I'm offering you information and inviting you to make your own choice. But I will tell you this with complete conviction: the Energy Restoration Protocol works. Not sometimes. Not for some people. But consistently, reliably, across diverse circumstances and populations.

If you implement it with genuine commitment, you will experience transformation. Your health will improve. Your energy will increase. Your body will heal. Your life will change.

I know this because I've lived it. Because I've seen it. Because science supports it. Because thousands of people have proven it.

The question now is what will you do with this information?

Final Words Before You Begin

You are reading this because some part of you knows that health is important. Some part of you is curious whether things could be different. Some part of you is ready for change.

Trust that part of you. It's wise. It's speaking the truth.

As you read this manifesto, remember you have power. More power than you realize. The power to change your health. The power to reverse disease. The power to create the future you want.

In Nature We Trust is not just a philosophy; it's a practical framework for claiming that power and using it to transform your life.

I'm honored to share this with you.

Welcome to the Energy Restoration Protocol.

Welcome home to health.

In Nature We Trust.

Life is Energy and Energy is Life.

—AXAY SHAH

DISCLAIMER

Important Notice

This manifesto is based on the author's personal over sixteen years of documented health transformation. It is *not* intended as medical advice or a substitute for professional medical care.

Before implementing any significant dietary or lifestyle changes, consult with your health care provider and share this manifesto. This is especially important if you have existing health conditions, take medications, are pregnant or breastfeeding, or have mental health conditions.

Individual results vary. While the Energy Restoration Protocol has supported health transformation for many people, not everyone will experience the same outcomes or timeline. Your unique circumstances, genetics, medical history, medications, and lifestyle factors all influence your results.

Work *with* your medical team, not against it. This manifesto is designed to complement, not replace, professional medical care. If you're on medications, work with your health care provider before making changes; medications may need adjustment as your health improves.

The author is not a licensed physician, registered dietitian, or medical professional. This manifesto reflects personal experience, scientific understanding of energy system dysfunction, and not clinical trials or peer-reviewed research.

You are responsible for your own health choices. By reading and implementing anything in this manifesto, you assume full responsibility for your decisions and outcomes.

If you have questions or concerns about implementing this protocol for your specific situation, consult a qualified health care provider who is familiar with plant-based nutrition and energy restoration principles.

Trust nature. Trust your body. Trust your medical team. Trust yourself.

One with Nature

I am one with all of nature,
You are one with all of nature.
From nowhere, we're bound to nature,
In colors and spirit, we've found our nature.
Divine honey, magic mushrooms call,
The universe dances, a cosmic song for all.
A butterfly floats through infinity's embrace,
Swimming in seas, I am the sea's face.
Leap in the playground, embrace the ride,
We're part of the universe, with nature as our guide.
Celestial symphonies in sheer silence play,
Emotions rise as chirping fills the day.
Gliding in love with the essence of nature,
From birth to death, life's eternal stature.
Life is nature, nature is life,
A timeless bond, free of strife.

—AXAY SHAH, "Bachu"

Philosophical Foundation

*Understanding Energy as
the Root of All Health*

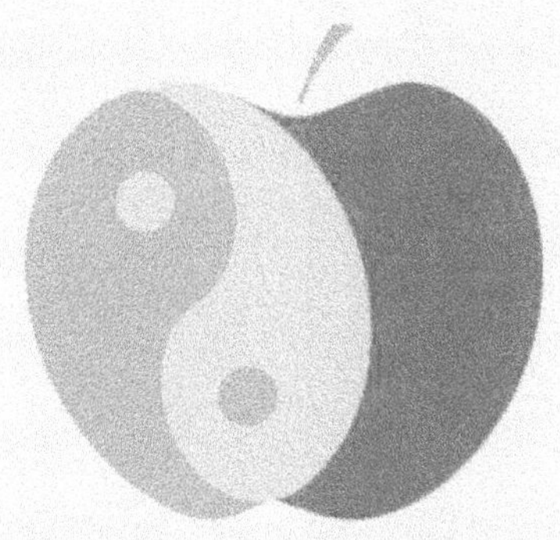

1

LIFE IS ENERGY AND ENERGY IS LIFE

The Energy Continuum: From First Breath to Last

There is a simple biological truth that contains profound meaning: From the moment you are born, your body begins producing energy. Your mitochondria begin their work. Energy (ATP—adenosine triphosphate) production begins. Life begins.

From that moment forward, for every second of your existence, your cells are producing energy. While you sleep, your mitochondria work. While you eat, your mitochondria work. While you exercise, while you rest, while you dream, your mitochondria never stop producing the energy that keeps you alive.

And when your mitochondria stop producing ATP, life ends.

Your entire life from birth to this present moment to your final breath is an energy-making process. Every moment you are alive, you are producing energy. Every moment you are alive, your body is choosing will this energy be abundant or depleted? Will this energy support health and vitality, or will it support only basic survival?

This understanding reframes everything. You are not a person who happens to have a metabolism. You are energy. You are an energy-producing system. Your health is determined by the quality and quantity of energy your cells produce. Your disease is determined by the insufficiency of that energy production.

From your first breath to your last, you are energy.

The question is: What kind of energy are you producing?

CONSIDER THIS MOMENT

Consider this moment, your heart beats. Your lungs breathe. Your eyes process these words. Trillions of cells in your body coordinate in perfect synchronization.

You think, feel, move, and dream. Your body repairs itself while you sleep. You heal from wounds. You digest food and transform it into blood, bone, and thought.

All of this, every function of your living body, is energy.

Not metaphorically. Not poetically. Biochemically, literally, measurably. Life is energy and energy is life.

This is not new information. Physics has understood this for centuries. Biology has documented it for decades. Yet, this simple truth remains perhaps the most misunderstood principle in medicine, nutrition, and health. We speak of disease as though it were a collection of separate problems; diabetes is one thing, heart disease another, Alzheimer's yet another. We prescribe medications targeting specific symptoms. We manage conditions. We accept illness as an inevitable part of aging.

But what if we're looking at this wrong?

What if all these seemingly separate diseases are actually expressions of the same fundamental problem? What if the root cause of virtually all chronic disease is not genetics or bad luck or aging itself, but rather a disruption of the energy system that keeps us alive?

And what if the solution is as simple as restoring that energy system?

This is the premise of this book. This is the framework that will transform how you understand your body, your health, and your power to heal.

Life is energy. Your health exists on a spectrum of energy availability. Your disease exists on a spectrum of energy dysfunction. Understanding this changes everything.

THE FUNDAMENTAL CURRENCY: ATP

At the foundation of every living cell exists a molecule called adenosine triphosphate (ATP). ATP is the energy currency of life. It is how your cells work, how they contract, communicate, synthesize proteins, repair damage, eliminate toxins, and maintain the intricate balance of life itself.

Your body produces roughly your body weight in ATP every single day.[1] Not once in your lifetime, every day. A 150-pound person produces 150 pounds of ATP daily, then breaks it down and rebuilds it constantly. Your cells cannot store ATP; they must produce it continuously, moment by moment, as long as you live.

This is not theoretical. This is happening in your body right now, at this very instant, in trillions of cells simultaneously.

Where is ATP made? In structures called mitochondria, the powerhouses of your cells. These remarkable organelles sit within each cell like tiny energy factories, consuming nutrients and oxygen and producing ATP. This process, called cellular respiration, is the foundation of all human life.[2]

When mitochondria function optimally, your cells have abundant ATP. When mitochondria do not function properly,[3] ATP production drops. When ATP drops, cells cannot maintain themselves. They deteriorate. They malfunction. They die or become dysfunctional.

This is where disease begins.

THE SPECTRUM OF ENERGY AND ORGAN VULNERABILITY

Health is not a binary state. You are not either healthy or sick. Instead, health exists on a spectrum determined by your energy status.

At one end of this spectrum is optimal energy availability. When your cells produce abundant ATP, they function beautifully. You have energy. You think clearly. You sleep well. You recover from exercise quickly. You fight off infections easily. You feel vital, alive, capable. You have capacity.

As you move along this spectrum toward lower energy availability, subtle changes begin. You notice fatigue that sleep doesn't fully resolve. Your mind feels slightly foggy. You catch colds more easily. You recover more slowly from exercise. You feel somewhat flat emotionally. You are still functioning, but at a lower capacity.

Continue further down the spectrum and the changes become more obvious. Fatigue becomes persistent and limiting. Brain fog becomes noticeable cognitive difficulty. You develop persistent pain or inflammation. Your mood shifts. You gain weight despite eating less. Your blood pressure rises. Your digestion becomes problematic. You develop pre-diabetes or early diabetes markers.

Continue further and disease becomes obvious. Full Type 2 diabetes. Heart disease. Cognitive decline. Chronic pain syndromes. Multiple medications become necessary.

But here is the critical insight, all of these conditions from subtle fatigue all the way to serious chronic disease exist on the same spectrum. They all reflect the same underlying problem: insufficient ATP production.

Yet there is another layer of complexity worth understanding, not all organs fail equally when ATP production drops. Different organs have vastly different energy demands, and they fail in predictable patterns based on those demands.

Your brain uses approximately 20 percent of your body's energy at rest, despite representing only 2 percent of your body weight.[4] The brain is extraordinarily energy hungry. When energy becomes scarce, the brain may be among the first to show dysfunction; hence, this is why brain fog, depression, and cognitive decline often appear early in the energy-depletion spectrum.

Your heart is even more demanding. This muscle contracts roughly one hundred thousand times daily. It never rests. The heart uses about 25 percent of your body's energy at rest. When energy becomes insufficient, the heart struggles to maintain its powerful, consistent contractions. Arrhythmias may develop. Heart function may decline. In some people, heart disease becomes their primary expression of energy system failure.

Your pancreas must produce constant insulin to manage blood glucose. When you eat, blood glucose rises, and the beta cells of the pancreas must respond with precise insulin secretion. This requires enormous ATP.[5] For people who consume refined carbohydrates and cause constant glucose spikes, the pancreas is under relentless ATP demand. Eventually it exhausts. The result: Type 2 diabetes becomes the primary expression of energy system failure.[6]

Your liver performs over 500 distinct functions, many of them ATP-intensive. Your muscles constantly require ATP for contraction and maintenance. Your immune system requires ATP to create antibodies and fight infections. Your DNA repair mechanisms require ATP to maintain your genome. Your detoxification systems require ATP to eliminate toxins.

The point is when ATP production becomes insufficient, different organs fail in different people depending on their individual vulnerabilities, their genetic predispositions, and their particular life stressors. A person with a family history of heart disease may develop cardiovascular failure first. A person with high insulin demand may develop diabetes first. A person with genetic vulnerabilities in brain energy metabolism may develop cognitive decline first.

But the underlying mechanism is identical in all cases: insufficient ATP production. The mitochondria are not making enough energy for cells to maintain themselves and perform their functions.

This understanding is profoundly important because it explains why the same intervention restoring mitochondrial energy production helps people with seemingly different diseases. You are not fixing diabetes. You are not fixing heart disease. You are restoring energy production, and as energy becomes available, whichever organs were energy starved begin to function properly again.

Mitochondrial Damage Cascade: How the System Breaks Down

To understand how to restore the energy system, you must understand how it breaks down. The process is not random. It follows a predictable cascade.

When you consume refined carbohydrates like white bread, white rice, or pasta, sugar glucose enters your bloodstream rapidly. Blood glucose spikes. Your pancreas detects the spike and releases insulin. Insulin signals cells to take up glucose. But because glucose enters so rapidly, cells absorb more than they need. Inside the cells, excess glucose is converted to triglycerides and stored as fat.[7]

This acute event is manageable. But when this pattern repeats refined carbohydrates at breakfast, lunch, dinner, and snacks, the cascade begins.

Repeated glucose spikes cause hyperinsulinemia, which is chronically elevated insulin levels. High insulin creates several problems simultaneously. First, constant high insulin drives fat storage, particularly visceral fat around your organs. Second, persistent high insulin causes cells to become desensitized to insulin signals; they literally stop responding. This is insulin resistance. Third, high insulin suppresses glucagon, the hormone that tells your body to access stored energy. Even though you have abundant fat stores, your body cannot access them for energy. You remain hungry despite being full of stored energy.

More critically for the energy system, during these glucose spikes, something destructive happens at the mitochondrial level. High glucose and high insulin together generate free radicals, unstable molecules that damage cellular structures. These free radicals attack the mitochondrial membranes. They damage the proteins that comprise the electron transport chain, the machinery that produces ATP. Oxidative stress increases. The mitochondria become damaged.

Simultaneously, high glucose creates advanced glycation end products (AGEs) through a process called glycation. Glucose molecules attach to proteins, creating sticky compounds that cross-link and damage cellular structures. The mitochondria are particular targets of this damage. The damage accumulates. Mitochondrial function deteriorates further.

Additionally, refined carbohydrates and processed foods lack the magnesium, chromium, and other minerals required as cofactors in energy production. Without these cofactors, even when fuel is available, the mitochondria cannot process it efficiently. ATP production drops further.

Meanwhile, industrial seed oils for instance, soybean, corn, canola) accumulate in cell membranes and mitochondrial membranes. These oxidized polyunsaturated fats are incorporated into the very structure of your cells. They make the membranes inflexible and permeable. Mitochondrial function deteriorates. Calcium leaks into cells when it shouldn't. Cells activate their death programs. More mitochondria are lost.

Simultaneously, damaged mitochondria produce excessive free radicals. Free radicals damage other mitochondria. One damaged mitochondrion triggers damage in others. The problem cascades. Mitochondrial density decreases. Surviving mitochondria are damaged. ATP production collapses.

Additionally, processed foods damage the gut lining. Additives, emulsifiers, and the absence of fiber compromise the intestinal barrier. The gut becomes permeable. Lipopolysaccharides (LPS) from bacterial cell walls leak through the damaged barrier into the bloodstream. These LPS molecules trigger systemic inflammation. Inflammation damages mitochondria throughout the body.

Over months and years of repeated refined carbohydrate consumption, industrial seed oil accumulation, and processed food damage to the gut, the cascade accelerates. Mitochondrial dysfunction becomes severe. ATP production becomes insufficient. Cells cannot maintain themselves. Tissue function declines. Symptoms appear. Disease emerges.

This is not sudden. This is not mysterious. This is a predictable cascade caused by the specific foods modern humans consume.

THE ENERGY BANKRUPTCY METAPHOR

Understanding the energy cascade requires understanding what happens when cells go bankrupt energetically.

Think of ATP as currency. Your cells are economic systems. They have income (ATP production) and expenses (energy required for all cellular functions). When income exceeds expenses, you have surplus. Cells can maintain themselves, repair damage, fight infections, maintain brain function, manage emotions, think clearly, and feel vital.

But what happens when income drops? What happens when ATP production declines while energy expenses remain constant?

Initially, cells draw down reserves. They have some capacity to store energy temporarily. But this reserve is small and depletes quickly. Within hours of reducing ATP production, reserves are depleted.

Then what? The cell must ration energy. It must prioritize which functions receive available ATP.

The brain gets priority. Survival depends on the brain maintaining consciousness and vital functions. If brain ATP drops too low, you die. So the brain gets the first claim on available ATP.

The heart gets priority. It must keep beating. If heart ATP drops too low, the heart fails and you die. So the heart maintains its energy demand.

The immune system gets priority. Survival depends on fighting infections. Immune cells require ATP to create antibodies and kill pathogens.

But other functions are not essential for immediate survival. Muscle maintenance is deferred. Tissue repair is deferred. Hormone production is reduced. Sex drive diminishes (reproduction is not essential for immediate survival). Cognitive functions beyond immediate survival are diminished. Memory, learning, mood regulation these are rationed.

This is why energy-depleted people experience cognitive decline. Not because their brains are broken, but because ATP has been rationed away from cognitive functions toward survival functions.

This is why energy-depleted people lose interest in activities they previously enjoyed. Not because of laziness or depression alone, but because the brain has rationed ATP away from reward-related functions.

This is why energy-depleted people have reduced libido. Not because there is a specific hormone deficiency, but because reproduction consumes ATP, and when energy is rationed, reproductive function is deprioritized.

This is why energy-depleted people gain weight despite eating less and exercising more. The body has entered energy conservation mode. Fat storage is prioritized over fat mobilization. Metabolism is suppressed. The body is trying to preserve energy for survival.

The cascade becomes downward spiraling. As ATP production drops, cells cannot repair themselves effectively. Damaged mitochondria accumulate. Energy production drops further. More rationing occurs. More symptoms emerge. More disease develops.

This is energy bankruptcy. And it is entirely predictable and reversible when you restore ATP production.

SYMPTOMS ARE NOT THE PROBLEM

Medicine has taught us to think of symptoms as the problem. A person develops high blood pressure, and the problem is defined as "high blood pressure." A person develops elevated blood glucose, and the problem is "diabetes." A person develops depression, and the problem is "depression."

But what if symptoms are not the problem? What if symptoms are the body's response to a deeper problem, the signal of energy bankruptcy?

Consider fatigue. When you feel persistently tired despite adequate sleep, your body is telling you that your cells do not have adequate ATP. Fatigue is the signal. The low ATP production is the problem. Treating the fatigue with stimulants like caffeine and medications mask the signal but does nothing to restore ATP production. You feel less tired, but your cells are still energy starved. The underlying problem persists and typically worsens.

Consider depression. When you feel persistently low in mood and lack motivation, your brain is telling you that your neurons do not have adequate ATP. Depression is the signal of energy bankruptcy in reward-related brain regions. Depression medication may increase neurotransmitters, but if ATP production remains low, the fundamental problem persists. The medication masks the symptom; it does not restore energy. And when the medication wears off or the brain adapts to it, the symptom returns because the energy problem remains.

Consider high blood pressure. When your blood pressure is elevated, your cardiovascular system is telling you the blood vessels cannot relax properly because the cells maintaining blood vessel function do not have adequate ATP. Blood pressure medication may lower the number, but if ATP production remains low, the underlying dysfunction persists. The vessels are still dysfunctional; the medication just forces them into a lower pressure state through chemical manipulation rather than healing.

Consider pain and inflammation. Pain is the signal of tissue damage or cellular distress. When you have chronic pain, your body is telling you tissues are damaged, ATP production is insufficient for repair, and the cells are in distress. Taking pain medication masks the signal. The tissue damage and ATP insufficiency remain. The pain returns when medication wears off.

Consider weight gain. Weight gain is the body's response to energy dysregulation. When ATP production is insufficient, the body increases fat storage as an attempt to preserve energy in more stable form. Weight loss medications and calorie restriction attempt to force weight down through external manipulation. But if ATP production remains low, the body fights back. Hunger increases. Metabolism decreases. Weight returns.

This is not to say symptoms don't matter or that medications are never appropriate during acute crises. But it is to say that treating symptoms without addressing the underlying energy dysfunction is fundamentally incomplete medicine. It is like treating a bank account's overdraft fees without addressing the fact that spending exceeds income. The fees keep getting paid, but the account never becomes solvent.

The breakthrough comes when you understand this: restore ATP production to optimal levels, and the body naturally corrects these symptoms because the root problem is addressed.

HOW MODERN FOOD DISRUPTS ENERGY PRODUCTION

The modern food system has fundamentally disrupted human energy production through multiple mechanisms.

First, refined carbohydrates cause glucose to enter the bloodstream too rapidly. This creates massive insulin spikes and the cascade of mitochondrial damage described above. Repeated insulin spikes damage mitochondria and create insulin resistance, the fundamental metabolic problem underlying Type 2 diabetes and the precursor to virtually all chronic disease.

Second, industrial seed oils contain oxidized polyunsaturated fats. During extraction and processing, these oils are heated, exposed to solvents, and chemically altered. Oxidation products form. These damaged fats accumulate in cell membranes and mitochondrial membranes when consumed. This accumulation impairs membrane function, increases free radical production, and damages mitochondrial structure. Oxidative stress increases. ATP production decreases.

Third, processed foods lack the micronutrients and phytonutrients required for optimal mitochondrial function. Magnesium, chromium, polyphenols, antioxidants, these compounds are either removed during processing or never present in processed foods. Without them, the mitochondria cannot function optimally. ATP production declines. The damage cascade accelerates.

Additionally, modern processed foods contain additives, emulsifiers, preservatives, and artificial sweeteners that damage the gut lining and promote systemic inflammation. Emulsifiers literally alter the mucus layer protecting your intestinal cells. The tight junctions between intestinal cells become leaky. Bacterial lipopolysaccharides cross the damaged barrier into the bloodstream. These trigger systemic inflammation, which damages mitochondria throughout the body.

The result is predictable: a population eating modern processed foods experiences epidemic rates of chronic disease. Not because of bad luck or genetics or aging, but because the modern food system disrupts mitochondrial function and ATP production in ways that create energy deficit in the cells.

The statistics bear this out starkly. In populations eating traditional plant-based raw food, Type 2 diabetes is rare, heart disease is rare, cognitive decline is rare. In populations that have adopted the modern processed-food diet, these diseases have become epidemic within a single generation. Not a slow genetic drift over centuries. A rapid shift within years. This is not about genetics. This is about energy system disruption from poor nutrition.

HOW NATURAL FOODS RESTORE ENERGY PRODUCTION

In contrast, plant-based raw foods, vegetables, fruits, legumes, whole grains, nuts, seeds, provide complete nutritional packages that restore and optimize mitochondrial function.

Whole plant foods contain abundant polyphenols. Over eight thousand different types of polyphenols exist in plant foods,[8] each with specific biological actions. Polyphenols are not vitamins you need in trace amounts. They are bioactive compounds that communicate with your cells, telling them what to do.

Polyphenols cross the blood-brain barrier and directly activate genes involved in mitochondrial biogenesis, the creation of new mitochondria. They activate sirtuins, a class of proteins involved in energy metabolism and longevity. They increase AMPK activity, an enzyme that regulates cellular energy status and tells cells to activate energy-producing pathways. In effect, polyphenols tell your cells to make more and better mitochondria.

Whole plant foods contain the full spectrum of vitamins and minerals required as cofactors in ATP production. Magnesium (required for over 300 enzymatic reactions), chromium (required for glucose tolerance factor), zinc (required for insulin synthesis), iron (required for electron transport), B vitamins (required for every step of energy production) all are abundant in whole plant foods, all are required for optimal ATP production. Without these cofactors, mitochondria cannot function efficiently. With them, optimal function is restored.

Whole plant foods contain fiber. Fiber feeds beneficial bacteria in your gut microbiome. These bacteria produce short-chain fatty acids, particularly butyrate, which reduces systemic inflammation, heals the gut lining, and directly supports mitochondrial function. Additionally, the integrity of the gut barrier is maintained, preventing the bacterial LPS leakage that triggers systemic inflammation.

Whole plant foods contain enzymes. Raw plant foods contain living enzymes that facilitate digestion and nutrient absorption. These enzymes remain active in your digestive system, reducing the work your digestive enzymes must perform and allowing more ATP to be available for other cellular functions.

The result is profound. When you consume whole plant foods, your mitochondria receive quality fuel, the supporting nutrients needed to process that fuel efficiently, and the signaling compounds that activate mitochondrial repair and regeneration.

ATP production optimizes. Energy becomes abundant. Cells function beautifully. Energy bankruptcy is reversed.

Your Power and Agency: The Choice That Changes Everything

Here is a truth that conventional medicine rarely emphasizes, and which changes everything about your relationship to your health: You created this energy deficit through choices. Specifically, through food choices.

If you consume refined carbohydrates, industrial seed oils, and processed foods, you are actively disrupting your mitochondrial function. You are creating the energy deficit that causes disease. This is not passive. This is active damage you are doing to your cells through the choices you make multiple times every day.

But here is the liberating corollary: if you created the energy deficit through your choices, you can reverse it through different choices.

This is not about willpower or self-blame. It is about understanding your power.

Conventional medicine teaches passive victimhood. You have diabetes because of your genes. You have heart disease because of bad luck. You have depression because of brain chemistry. These narratives remove agency. They position you as a victim of circumstances beyond your control. You must take medications. You must accept your disease. You must manage it for life.

But this is not accurate. While genetics influence your predispositions, they do not determine your fate. Genes express themselves based on environmental signals. The primary environmental signal determining whether genetic predispositions activate or remain dormant is nutrition. The foods you choose activate or deactivate genetic predispositions toward disease.

In populations eating traditional plant-based whole foods, people with the same genetic predispositions remain healthy. The genes do not express as disease because the nutritional environment does not activate them.

In populations eating processed foods, the same genetic predispositions activate and express as disease because the nutritional environment activates them.

The difference is not genetics. The difference is choice.

This is profoundly empowering. It means you have control. It means your health is not determined by fate or genetics or bad luck. It is determined by the choices you make, multiple times every day, about what you eat.

Every apple you choose instead of apple juice is a choice to restore your energy system. Every meal of whole plant foods is a choice to heal your mitochondria. Every time you choose not to consume processed foods is a choice to stop actively poisoning your cells.

These are not small choices. These are powerful choices. These choices, accumulated day after day, month after month, transform your health.

And here is what makes this even more powerful, once you make these choices consistently, you see results. Your energy improves. Your symptoms diminish. Your blood work normalizes. You feel better. The positive feedback is immediate and obvious. Your body responds almost immediately to being given what it needs.

This is why people stick with this approach long term. Not because of discipline or willpower, but because the results are so undeniable that returning to previous eating patterns loses all appeal. Once you experience how good you feel with abundant ATP production, the foods that created the energy deficit lose their power to tempt you.

Your health is not something that happens to you. Your health is something you create one choice at a time, one meal at a time.

You have power. The question is: Will you use it?

SYMPTOMS RESOLVE: DISEASE REVERSES

When you restore your energy system, something remarkable happens. The body's own healing capacity emerges.

Symptoms that seemed permanent begin to resolve. Fatigue lifts as ATP production increases. Cognitive fog clears as the brain receives abundant energy. Mood elevates. Inflammation decreases. Weight normalizes. Blood glucose normalizes. Blood pressure normalizes. Cholesterol improves. Digestion improves. Sleep improves.

These are not coincidences. These are inevitable consequences of restoring energy production to optimal levels. When cells have abundant ATP, they do what they evolved to do—maintain themselves, repair damage, and function beautifully.

This has been demonstrated thousands of times. People with Type 2 diabetes for twenty years achieve completely normal blood glucose within months of restoring their energy systems through plant-based whole food nutrition. People with heart disease experience plaque regression. People with depression experience mood restoration. People with cognitive decline experience cognitive improvement.

These are not miracles or exceptions. These are predictable results of restoring mitochondrial function.

YOUR BODY'S EXTRAORDINARY HEALING CAPACITY

Here is perhaps the most important truth in this entire framework: your body is not broken. Your body is not fundamentally defective. Your body is supremely intelligent and possesses remarkable healing capacity.

When you are diagnosed with Type 2 diabetes, you are not learning that your body is incapable of managing blood glucose. You are learning that your mitochondria have been so damaged by poor nutrition that they cannot produce the ATP required for normal glucose regulation. But the blueprint for normal glucose regulation is still encoded in your cells. The machinery is still there. It is just energy starved.

Restore that energy, and the system functions again.

When you experience depression or anxiety or cognitive fog, you are not learning that your brain is fundamentally broken. You are learning that your neurons are energy starved and cannot produce the neurotransmitters or maintain the connections required for optimal mood and cognition. Restore energy to those neurons, and your mood and cognition normalize.

When you develop heart disease or high blood pressure, you are not learning that your cardiovascular system is fundamentally defective. You are learning that your vascular endothelium and cardiac muscle are energy starved and cannot perform their functions. Restore that energy, and your cardiovascular function improves.

The profound and liberating insight when understanding health through an energy lens is that your body does not want to be sick. Your body wants to be healthy. Disease is not an inevitable outcome. Disease is a consequence of energy deprivation. Restore the energy, and the body naturally returns to health.

The Vision Forward

This book is built on this framework. Every chapter that follows is grounded in the understanding that life is energy, health is energy optimization, disease is energy dysfunction, and the solution is energy restoration through alignment with nature's design for human nutrition.

This is not a complicated concept, though implementing it requires commitment. This is not new science, though it represents a paradigm shift from conventional medicine's disease-focused model. This is not theory; it is backed by decades of research and demonstrated by millions of people who have transformed their health by understanding and applying this principle.

The chapters ahead will take you deeper into this framework. You will understand the specific mechanisms by which natural foods restore energy. You will see how the same protocol addresses multiple diseases. You will learn the practical steps to restore your energy system. You will hear stories of people who have recovered their health by applying these principles.

But before all of that, understand this foundational truth: Your body is designed for health. You are not broken. Your cells are supremely intelligent. You possess extraordinary healing capacity. You have power over your health. Your choices matter.

What you lack is not capacity. What you lack is energy.

Restore that energy through alignment with natural nutrition, and your body will do what it evolved to do: heal, thrive, and express vitality.

From your first breath to your last, you are energy.

Life is energy.

Energy is life.

Restore your energy, and you restore your life.

2

THE MODERN DISCONNECTION

The Evolutionary Mismatch

Your body is not designed for the food it is eating.

This simple statement contains a profound truth that explains the disease epidemic sweeping the modern world. Your body, your digestive system, your metabolism, your mitochondria, your entire biological machinery evolved over millions of years to process and thrive on specific foods.

Plants. Whole plants. Vegetables, fruits, legumes, nuts, seeds, and whole grains in their natural, intact form. These are the foods humans evolved to consume. Archaeological evidence, anthropological studies, and comparative anatomy all point to the same conclusion: humans are fundamentally plant-eaters. We are herbivores by evolutionary design, with some capacity to eat animal products opportunistically, but with our entire digestive and metabolic system optimized for plant-based whole foods.

For hundreds of thousands of years, the vast majority of human evolution, humans ate these foods. We ate plants in the forms they grew. We ate fruits with seeds and skin intact. We ate vegetables with fiber and nutrients preserved. We ate legumes after soaking and cooking. We ate nuts and seeds raw. We ate whole grains when we could access them. We never ate refined carbohydrates. We never ate extracted oils. We never consumed processed foods with additives and preservatives.

Our bodies adapted to this diet at every level. Our teeth are designed to chew fibrous plant foods. Our digestive system is designed to ferment fiber. Our microbiome evolved to process plant foods. Our metabolic pathways are optimized for plant-based nutrition. Our mitochondria developed their energy-producing machinery on the fuel plant foods provide.

We became human on this diet.

And then 150 years ago, in the blink of an eye in evolutionary time, everything changed.

THE 150-YEAR ABERRATION

One hundred and fifty years is not long. In evolutionary terms, it is nothing. Your genes have not changed substantially in 150 years. Your digestive system has not adapted. Your metabolic machinery has not evolved. Your mitochondria have not developed new capacities.

Yet in these 150 years, the food humans eat has undergone a radical transformation.

The Industrial Revolution of the 1800s triggered the Agricultural Revolution, which triggered the Processed Food Revolution. Suddenly, humans had the technology to refine grains, extract oils, process foods, preserve them with chemicals, and distribute them globally. Suddenly, foods that previously required hours of preparation could be made instantly. Suddenly, foods that were seasonal became available year-round. Suddenly, the human food supply was dominated by foods our bodies had never encountered.

This was not a gradual shift. This was a radical discontinuity. Within a few decades, processed foods went from nonexistent to dominant in industrialized populations. Within a century, they became the primary food source. Within 150 years, processed foods have become so normalized that most people have never eaten food the way humans ate it for the preceding hundreds of thousands of years.

Your great-grandmother likely ate primarily whole foods. Your grandmother may have started consuming some processed foods. Your parents ate a mixed diet. You were likely raised on predominantly processed foods. Your children may have never eaten a truly whole food diet.

In just three generations, humans disconnected from the foods we evolved to eat and adopted foods our bodies had no evolutionary preparation for.

What Changed 150 Years Ago:
The Timeline of Disconnection

To understand how we lost our way, you must understand the specific transformations that occurred in the food supply.

BEFORE 1870: THE WORLD YOUR GREAT-GRANDPARENTS KNEW

Imagine your kitchen in 1860. No refrigerator. No electricity. No packaged foods. No supermarkets.

Your great-grandmother prepared meals from what was available locally and seasonally. Winter meant root vegetables stored in cellars, dried beans and legumes from fall harvest, preserved vegetables fermented in brine. Spring meant fresh greens and early vegetables. Summer meant an abundance of berries, stone fruits, vegetables ripening in gardens. Fall meant harvest preservation with canning, fermenting, drying.

Grains were whole grains. Flour was ground from whole wheat berries at the local mill. Bread was made at home from this flour, risen with naturally occurring yeasts, baked fresh. Rice was brown rice with its nutrient-rich bran intact. Oats were rolled by hand, not instant-processed. Sugar was available but expensive; honey was more common and used sparingly.

Meat was occasional, not daily. Perhaps a chicken on Sunday. Perhaps fish if you lived near water. Perhaps game if you hunted. Dairy was fresh milk from local cows, used to make cheese and butter. But the foundation of every meal was vegetables, grains, and legumes.

A typical meal would be a thick vegetable and legume soup, dark whole grain bread, maybe some cheese. Or a grain-based porridge with vegetables and legumes. Or baked root vegetables with herbs. Simple. Whole. Nourishing.

There were no packaged foods. No refined carbohydrates. No extracted oils. No chemical additives or preservatives. Food came from plants and animals in forms that required preparation, but once prepared, nourished the body completely.

1870–1900: THE FIRST TRANSFORMATION WHEN REFINED GRAINS ARRIVE

Then came the technology that changed everything: mechanical grain refinement.

Before 1870, refining grain was labor intensive. The nutrient-rich bran and germ had to be manually removed from wheat berries, a process that was expensive and not widely done. White flour was a luxury food, affordable only to the wealthy.

In 1870, steam-powered grain mills were developed. Suddenly, white flour could be produced cheaply and at scale. Within decades, white flour became the dominant grain product.

The implications were profound. White flour lasts longer than whole grain flour (the bran and germ contain oils that go rancid). White flour could be shipped long distances without spoiling. White flour was whiter, which was associated with purity and luxury. Food manufacturers and millers loved white flour. It was profitable, storable, and marketable.

But white flour is nutritionally devastated. The bran contains fiber, minerals, and B vitamins. The germ contains healthy fats and more nutrients. Remove these, and what remains is mostly starch carbohydrates without supporting nutrients.

Suddenly, by 1890, white bread had become the norm in developing nations. Whole grain bread, once the universal standard, became associated with poverty. White bread became the aspirational food of the middle class.

Your great-grandmother might have transitioned in this era. Perhaps she still baked bread at home from whole grain flour in her youth. But by middle age, she might have purchased white bread from a bakery, associating it with progress and modernity.

This single shift from whole grain to refined grain triggered the beginning of metabolic disruption. Refined carbohydrates began entering the food supply at scale. Glucose spikes became common. The first metabolic changes began occurring in populations consuming white bread.

1900–1920: SUGAR BECOMES ACCESSIBLE

Simultaneously, sugar production industrialized. Sugar cane and sugar beets, once labor intensive to process, became industrial commodities. Sugar production scaled up. Prices collapsed.

In 1800, the average person consumed about eight pounds of sugar per year. By 1900, it was twenty pounds per year. By 1920, it was forty pounds per year.[1]

This was revolutionary. For the first time in human history, sugar became an affordable, everyday food for the general population. Suddenly, foods that were previously impossible were possible: sweet bread, sweet pastries, sweet breakfast cereals, sweet everything.

Your grandmother grew up in an era when sugar was becoming normal. Her mother perhaps made jams and preserves, which required sugar. Her grandmother rarely made such foods; they were too expensive. But by your grandmother's childhood, the first sugar-sweetened breakfast cereals were being marketed as modern nutrition.

1920–1950: VEGETABLE OILS AND TRANS FATS TRANSFORM THE FOOD SUPPLY

The next transformation was the rise of extracted vegetable oils and the creation of trans fats.

Before 1920, fats in the food supply came primarily from whole foods: nuts, seeds, olives, avocados, and animal products. These were unrefined, whole foods containing the fat along with other nutrients.

In the 1920s, technology allowed the industrial extraction and hydrogenation of seed oils. Hydrogenation takes liquid vegetable oil and converts it into solid shortening through a chemical process that creates trans fats that do not exist in nature.

This technology was a triumph of food engineering. Vegetable shortening was cheaper than butter. It lasted longer without going rancid. It could be used in countless products. It was a manufacturer's dream.

By 1950, vegetable oils and trans fats had become the standard fats in commercial baking and food preparation. Your mother's generation grew up eating foods made with these artificial fats, margarine instead of butter, shortening instead of lard, refined vegetable oils instead of whole food fats.

The consequence was invisible but profound: oxidized polyunsaturated fats began accumulating in people's cell membranes and mitochondrial membranes. Cellular dysfunction began increasing. But the effect was subtle enough that it took decades to manifest as an obvious disease.

1950–1970: THE PROCESSED FOOD EXPLOSION

After World War II, food technology exploded. Canning technology advanced. Freezing technology improved. Chemical preservation became sophisticated. Artificial colors, flavors, and preservatives proliferated.

For the first time, truly shelf-stable foods could be manufactured foods that would remain edible for months or years without spoiling. Convenience foods exploded: TV dinners, instant meals, packaged snacks, sugary cereals marketed to children.

Your parents' generation grew up with this food revolution. Their mothers increasingly used packaged convenience foods. Homemade meals became less common. Processed foods became more common. The shift was dramatic.

A meal that once required hours of preparation starting with whole ingredients could now be prepared by simply opening packages and heating.

But the nutritional cost was enormous. These processed foods were stripped of nutrients, loaded with refined carbohydrates and added sugars, filled with artificial additives, and made from refined seed oils.

The foundation of metabolic health was eroding rapidly.

1970–2000: THE DIET-DISEASE CONSPIRACY AND THE LOW-FAT RECOMMENDATION

Here is where the story becomes actively deceptive.

In the 1960s, research began showing a correlation between dietary fat and heart disease. The famous Seven Countries Study suggested that saturated fat consumption correlated with heart disease rates.

This research was not wrong, but it was incomplete. What the research actually showed was that processed foods high in saturated fat and refined carbohydrates correlated with heart disease. But the food industry seized on this research to promote a different narrative, all fat was bad, and refined carbohydrates were safe.

In 1977, the US government released dietary guidelines recommending a low-fat diet. The primary author of these guidelines was influenced by the sugar industry, which had funded research "proving" that sugar was safe and that fat was the problem.[2]

The result was that official government dietary recommendations shifted away from whole foods and toward low-fat, high-carbohydrate processed foods. Low-fat cookies replaced regular cookies. Low-fat snacks proliferated. Refined carbohydrates increased dramatically as fats were removed.

But here is what happened: people eating a low-fat diet didn't get healthier. They got sicker.

Why? Because when you remove fat from food, you remove satiety signals. People eating low-fat foods didn't feel satisfied. They ate more. They consumed more refined carbohydrates. Blood glucose spikes increased. Insulin spikes increased. Metabolic dysfunction accelerated.[3]

Additionally, the low-fat recommendation was based on incomplete science. The correlation between saturated fat and heart disease was real, but causation was more complex. Processed foods high in refined carbohydrates, industrial seed oils, and additives were the real culprit, not saturated fat from whole foods.

But by promoting the low-fat message, the food industry convinced the world to eat even more refined carbohydrates and even more processed foods.

Your generation grew up being told that low-fat was healthy. Parents bought low-fat snacks for their children, thinking they were being healthy. Schools served low-fat meals. The result was that metabolic dysfunction accelerated.

2000–PRESENT: ULTRAPROCESSED FOODS DOMINATE

Today, the modern food supply has reached its logical conclusion: ultraprocessed foods now represent the majority of calories consumed in developed nations.

A study by the National Institutes of Health found that ultraprocessed foods now represent 57.9 percent of calories consumed in the United States.[4] For children, it's even higher at 67 percent of calories coming from ultraprocessed foods.

These are not foods. These are products. They are engineered combinations of refined carbohydrates, extracted oils, added sugars, and chemical additives designed to maximize profit and encourage overeating.

Your children likely consume ultraprocessed foods at almost every meal, breakfast cereals laden with sugar and additives, packaged snacks engineered for maximum appeal, fast food meals designed by food scientists to override satiety signals, drinks loaded with high-fructose corn syrup or artificial sweeteners.

The disconnection is now complete. Most people have never eaten the foods their ancestors ate. Most children have never experienced the taste of truly whole food unmodified by processing.

The Disease Epidemic: The Timeline Is Not Coincidence

Now you must connect the dots. The food system timeline correlates perfectly with the disease epidemic timeline.

1870–1900: REFINED GRAINS INTRODUCED

Diabetes was rare. In 1880, Type 2 diabetes affected perhaps 1–2 percent of the population. Medical textbooks called it "diabetes mellitus," literally "honeyed urine disease" and classified it as a disease of the wealthy, affecting only those eating excessive rich foods.

But as refined grain consumption increased, something shifted.

1920–1950: REFINED CARBOHYDRATES AND TRANS FATS EXPLODE; HEART DISEASE EMERGES

In 1920, heart disease was not a leading cause of death. Autopsies of people who died from other causes showed clear arteries. Atherosclerosis was rare.

By 1950, heart disease had become the leading cause of death in developed nations.[5]

The timing is not a coincidence. The arrival of refined carbohydrates and trans fats preceded the heart disease epidemic by a specific lag time, the time required for metabolic dysfunction to manifest as arterial damage. Young people in the 1920s to 1930s began consuming processed foods in unprecedented quantities. By the 1950s, they were dying of heart disease at rates that were shocking.[6]

In 1950, heart disease killed approximately two hundred thousand Americans per year. Today, it kills over seven hundred thousand. The epidemic has not slowed; it has accelerated.

1950–1970: CANCER RATES RISE; DEMENTIA APPEARS

As processed foods became ubiquitous, cancer rates began increasing. Breast cancer, colon cancer, prostate cancer all showed rising trends starting in the 1950s.[7]

Similarly, dementia and Alzheimer's disease began appearing. Before 1950, dementia was uncommon. Your great-grandparents' generation rarely experienced cognitive decline if they lived to old age. Mentally sharp grandparents at eighty were common.

Today, cognitive decline in aging is so expected that it seems normal. We have normalized brain deterioration. We call it "senior moments" and expect it to be inevitable. We have built care facilities for dementia as though it were a natural part of aging.

It is not natural. It is a consequence of the modern food system.

1970–2000: DIABETES EXPLODES; OBESITY BECOMES EPIDEMIC

After the low-fat diet recommendations of 1977, something dramatic happened.

Diabetes rates exploded. Remember in 1900, perhaps 1–2 percent of the population had Type 2 diabetes. By 1950, it was 3–4 percent. But after 1977, the increase accelerated dramatically.

By 1980, diabetes increased to 5–6 percent of the population. By 1990, 7–8 percent. By 2000, 10–12 percent. By 2010, 15–18 percent. By 2020, 25–30 percent.[8]

Today, there are over 37 million Americans, with estimates suggesting 1 in 3 Americans will develop Type 2 diabetes in their lifetime, if current trends continue.

This is not a gradual increase. This is an explosive epidemic correlated precisely with the promotion of low-fat, high-refined-carbohydrate foods.

Simultaneously, obesity rates exploded. Before 1970, obesity was uncommon. Your great-grandparents' generation rarely saw obese people. It was a curiosity.

By 1980, perhaps 15 percent of Americans were obese. By 2000, it was 30 percent. Today, over 40 percent of Americans are obese, and childhood obesity rates are at historic highs.

This is not a coincidence with the low-fat diet recommendation. This is cause and effect.

2000–PRESENT: MENTAL HEALTH CRISIS; CHRONIC DISEASE EPIDEMIC

The twenty-first century has witnessed exploding rates of depression, anxiety, ADHD, and other mental health conditions.

Antidepressant medications have become among the most prescribed drugs in America. One in four women and one in ten men are currently taking antidepressants.

ADHD diagnoses have skyrocketed from rare to epidemic. Children are medicated for attention problems at rates that would be shocking to previous generations.

Anxiety disorders are now the most common mental health condition, affecting millions.

This is presented as a mental health crisis. But it correlates precisely with worsening food quality and increasing ultraprocessed food consumption.

Simultaneously, chronic disease rates have become staggering. Multiple chronic conditions are now common. A person with three or four chronic diseases requiring multiple medications is no longer unusual; it is becoming the norm.

Autoimmune diseases have become epidemic. Chronic pain syndromes have become epidemic. Digestive disorders have become epidemic. Allergies and asthma have become epidemic.

All correlate with the adoption of the modern food system.

The Specific Stories: How This Happened to Real People

Abstract statistics are less persuasive than real stories. So let me tell you stories.

THE OKINAWA STORY: HEALTH LOST IN A SINGLE GENERATION

The Okinawans of Japan represent one of the world's Blue Zones populations known for exceptional health and longevity. For centuries, Okinawans lived healthily into their nineties and beyond.

Their diet was distinctive: primarily sweet potatoes, vegetables, legumes, and grains. Meat was rare, perhaps eaten once monthly. Dairy was absent (no milk-drinking culture). Processed foods did not exist.

Medical researchers studying Okinawans in the 1950s documented remarkable health. Type 2 diabetes was virtually nonexistent. Heart disease was rare. Cancer rates were low. Obesity was absent. Mental health was robust. Cognitive decline in aging was uncommon.

An eighty-year-old Okinawan was typically energetic, mentally sharp, and physically capable.

Then, after World War II, American military presence introduced American processed foods. Convenience foods became available. Fast food appeared. Soft drinks arrived. Processed snacks proliferated.

The Okinawan population had a choice to maintain their traditional diet or adopt the new available foods. Some maintained tradition. Many adopted the new foods, especially younger generations who associated processed foods with modernity and American success.

The results were catastrophic.

Within one generation, literally twenty to thirty years, disease rates in Okinawa matched American disease rates.[9]

Type 2 diabetes became common. Heart disease appeared. Obesity became visible. Mental health problems emerged. Cognitive decline in aging became expected.

By the year 2000, an Okinawan population that had been among the healthiest on Earth became indistinguishable from the sick populations of developed Western nations.

The genetic population had not changed. The only change was food.

This is the power of the food system. This is what happens when a population disconnects from whole foods and adopts processed foods.

THE NATIVE AMERICAN STORY: DISEASE IN TWO GENERATIONS

Native Americans maintained health for thousands of years on traditional diets, plants, game, and fish, adapted to local ecosystems.

In the early to mid-1900s, Native Americans were forced onto reservations with limited access to traditional foods. Government-provided food aid consisted primarily of processed foods, refined grains, sugar, and cheap commodities.

The transition from traditional foods to processed foods happened rapidly, within a generation or two.

The health consequences were devastating.

Today, Native Americans have among the highest rates of Type 2 diabetes in the world. The Pima Indians have a diabetes rate of approximately 50 percent, meaning half the adult population has Type 2 diabetes.[10] This is not genetic predisposition; this is the food system's effect on a population that maintained health for thousands of years until they were forced to eat processed foods.

Other chronic diseases followed: heart disease, obesity, mental health disorders. Entire populations were devastated, not by any external force of nature, but by the food system imposed upon them.

This is the most dramatic example of how the modern food system creates disease in populations that were previously healthy.

YOUR FAMILY'S STORY: HOW YOUR GRANDPARENTS DISCONNECTED

Now let me tell you a story that is likely your story.

Your great-grandmother was probably born in the late 1800s or early 1900s. She grew up in a world without electricity, without refrigeration, without packaged foods. She likely grew vegetables in a garden. She likely preserved food for winter through fermentation and canning. She likely made bread at home. She likely didn't have access to processed foods, not because she was virtuous, but because they didn't exist.

Her health was probably decent, though medical care was limited. If she lived to old age, she probably remained relatively capable. Dementia was not expected. Chronic disease was not the default state of aging.

Your grandmother was born in the 1920s or 1930s. She grew up partly in the old world her mother knew, but increasingly in the new world of processed foods. She probably ate some whole foods her mother still cooked and still grew gardens. But increasingly, processed foods were available.

Her mother bought white bread from the bakery instead of baking at home. Her mother used canned vegetables. Her mother began buying packaged convenience foods. The transition was happening, but it wasn't complete.

Your grandmother probably developed her first chronic disease in her fifties or sixties. High blood pressure, perhaps. Or early heart disease. Or diabetes. These were becoming common but not yet universal.

Your mother was born in the 1940s or 1950s. By her childhood, the transition was complete. Her mother was using packaged convenience foods regularly. Whole grain bread was unusual. White bread was normal. Refined carbohydrates were the foundation of meals.

Your mother grew up with processed foods as the normal food supply. She probably had better health than your grandmother, antibiotics and modern medicine were more available. But she probably developed her first chronic disease in her forties or fifties. This was becoming normal for people in middle age with high blood pressure, heart disease, or diabetes was expected.

Your mother probably accepted this as inevitable. "Everyone gets something," people said. "It's just part of aging."

You were born in the 1960s–1980s. By your childhood, ultraprocessed foods dominated. Your parents probably bought low-fat snacks thinking they were healthy. Your school lunches were processed foods. Your after-school snacks were packaged processed foods.

If you had high blood pressure or elevated blood glucose in your thirties or forties, you probably accepted it as your genetic destiny. "My father had high blood pressure, so I'll have high blood pressure," you might have thought.

But this is not genetic destiny. This is the food system's effect across generations.

Your great-grandmother probably never had high blood pressure, she ate whole foods. Your grandmother developed it in her sixties because processed foods were becoming common. Your mother developed it in her fifties because processed foods were normal. You developed it in your forties because ultraprocessed foods are ubiquitous.

Each generation, the disease appears earlier and is more severe, not because of genetic changes, but because each generation consumes progressively more processed foods.

This is your family's story. This is most people's story.

THE SUGAR INDUSTRY DECEPTION: HOW WE WERE MANIPULATED

Now I must tell you a story about deception.

In the 1960s, internal documents from the sugar industry were discovered (through Freedom of Information Act requests) revealing deliberate manipulation of science.

The sugar industry knew that sugar was problematic for health. Internal research showed this. But rather than addressing the problem, the sugar industry decided to bury the research and manipulate public perception.[11]

They funded researchers to "prove" that fat, not sugar, was the problem. They influenced academic institutions through donations. They shaped dietary guidelines through lobbying and influence.

The result was the low-fat diet recommendation of 1977, which specifically directed people away from fat and toward refined carbohydrates (including sugar).

This was not an accidental policy. This was deliberate manipulation designed to protect sugar industry profits at the expense of public health.

The evidence is clear in declassified documents. Internal sugar industry communications show they knew what they were doing. They deliberately promoted false science to protect profits.

This deception led directly to the obesity and diabetes epidemics. Millions of people followed low-fat diet recommendations, consumed more refined carbohydrates and sugar, and developed chronic diseases as a result.

This is not a conspiracy theory. This is documented history.

THE KASPER MOMENT: GRANDMOTHER'S KITCHEN VS. YOUR KITCHEN

Let me tell you about a specific comparison that illustrates the disconnection.

Your grandmother's kitchen in 1950 probably looked like this: a stove (wood-burning or early gas), a counter space for food preparation, a few pots and pans, dried beans and grains in jars, fresh vegetables in a root cellar or cool pantry, fresh fruit in season, herbs hung to dry. Maybe twenty to thirty basic ingredients total.

She prepared food from these whole ingredients daily. A meal took hours to prepare. She made bread, soups, stews, and vegetable dishes. Everything from scratch.

Your kitchen today probably looks like this: electric stove, microwave, dishwasher, cabinets full of packaged processed foods, freezer full of frozen convenience meals, refrigerator with prepackaged items, maybe fresh produce that will spoil before being used.

Preparing a meal now takes minutes but involves mostly opening packages and heating them.

The contrast is stark. Your grandmother's kitchen was designed for whole food preparation. Your kitchen is designed for processed food consumption.

This is not progress. This is disconnection.

HOW PROCESSED FOODS DISRUPT THE ENERGY SYSTEM

At the mitochondrial level, processed foods disrupt energy production through the mechanisms described in Chapter 1. But it is worth revisiting them in the context of how radically different processed foods are from the foods humans evolved eating.

Refined carbohydrates cause massive glucose spikes unknown in human evolution. Your ancestors never consumed glucose that entered the bloodstream this rapidly. The pancreas responds with massive insulin spikes. The cascade of mitochondrial damage begins.

Industrial seed oils contain oxidized polyunsaturated fats that never existed in nature. Your ancestors never consumed rancid, oxidized oils. When these damaged fats accumulate in cell membranes, they damage the membrane structure that mitochondria depend on.

Processed foods lack the micronutrients whole foods contain. Your ancestors never consumed food that was nutritionally incomplete. Refined grain has had the mineral-rich germ and bran removed. Refined sugar provides only calories with no supporting nutrients. Processed foods are nutritional voids. Mitochondria cannot function optimally without the nutrients they require.

Food additives, emulsifiers, preservatives, artificial sweeteners never existed in human evolution. Your ancestors never consumed these compounds. When emulsifiers damage the gut lining, bacterial lipopolysaccharides trigger systemic inflammation that damages mitochondria throughout the body.

At every level, processed foods are evolutionarily foreign. They disrupt the energy production your body evolved to perform on whole plant foods.

Why Conventional Medicine Misses the Root Cause

Conventional medicine has failed to solve the chronic disease epidemic because it treats disease as the problem, rather than treating the underlying energy disruption as the problem.

A person develops Type 2 diabetes, and the medical response is to prescribe medication to lower blood glucose. A person develops heart disease, and the response is to prescribe medication to lower cholesterol or blood pressure. A person develops depression, and the response is to prescribe medication to modify neurotransmitters. A person develops arthritis, and the response is to prescribe medication to reduce inflammation.

All of this is treating symptoms while the root cause energy system disruption from processed foods continues unaddressed.

This is not a failure of individual doctors. Most doctors are compassionate and well-intentioned. **It is a failure of the system.** Medical education teaches disease management, not health optimization. Medical training focuses on pharmacology, not nutrition. Medical practice is structured around treating diseases as separate problems, not understanding diseases as expressions of a unified root cause.

Additionally, the food and pharmaceutical industries have shaped medical recommendations. The same industries that profit from selling processed foods profit from selling medications to treat diseases caused by those processed foods. There is no financial incentive to address the root cause. There is enormous financial incentive to manage symptoms with medications.

The result is chronic disease continues to increase despite medication use increasing. More people take more medications, yet disease rates rise. This is predictable when you are treating symptoms without addressing the root cause.

Why We Collectively Accepted the Disconnection

This raises a crucial question: How did humanity collectively abandon the foods we evolved to eat and adopt foods that damage our health? Why did this disconnection happen?

The answer is multifaceted.

First, the shift was gradual enough that it seemed normal. Your parents ate more processed food than their parents. You eat more than your parents. Your children eat more than you. At each step, the change seemed unremarkable. It was only across generations that the radical discontinuity became obvious.

Second, the food industry spent enormous resources marketing processed foods as modern, convenient, and desirable. Advertising created the association between processed foods and progress, sophistication, and success. Whole foods were positioned as old-fashioned and inferior.

Third, the food industry shaped medical and nutritional guidance through funding research and professional organizations. The low-fat diet recommendations that dominated from the 1970s forward were shaped by the sugar industry. Plant-based recommendations were suppressed in favor of recommendations favoring animal products and processed foods. Official dietary guidelines came to recommend processed foods as acceptable.

Fourth, processed foods were marketed and perceived as cheaper than whole foods. As food corporations industrialized and subsidized certain crops, processed foods were positioned as economically accessible to populations that could not afford fresh whole foods. For decades, this narrative that healthy eating requires expensive organic produce has been used to justify processed food consumption by low-income populations.

However, this narrative is demonstrably false. The Energy Restoration Protocol using whole plant foods (fruits, vegetables, seasonal produce, nuts, seeds) is substantially cheaper than processed foods when compared directly. The author has documented this reality: maintaining optimal health on plant-based raw foods costs approximately $5 per day, compared to the US average daily food spending of $25. This evidence is publicly documented in video format. Raw food is not a luxury; it is the most economically accessible path to health. Cost is not a legitimate barrier to implementing the Energy Restoration Protocol; this narrative has been weaponized to keep populations sick while consuming profitable processed foods.

Fifth, convenience was real. Whole food–based cooking is time consuming. Processed foods offered genuine convenience for busy modern life. The trade-off of health for convenience seemed like a reasonable choice in the moment, even though the long-term consequence was disease.

Sixth, the disconnection happened during a period of medical optimism. Antibiotics had recently been discovered and were saving lives. Vaccines were controlling infectious diseases. Medications were becoming more powerful. The belief emerged that medicine could handle whatever health problems arose. The idea that we should prevent disease through nutrition seemed unnecessary when medicine would fix any problems that appeared.

Seventh, there was genuine ignorance. For most people through most of this period, the connection between food and disease was not obvious. People did not understand mitochondrial dysfunction. They did not understand the mechanisms by which processed foods cause disease. They simply ate what was available and what advertising promoted.

All of these factors combined to create a collective disconnection from whole foods and acceptance of processed foods. It was not a deliberate choice to poison ourselves. It was a gradual, incremental process enabled by profit-driven food corporations, industry influence over science and medical recommendations, economic pressures on lower-income families, genuine convenience advantages of processed foods, and lack of understanding about the mechanisms by which food affects health.

The Reversal: It Is Possible

But here is the crucial point: this disconnection is recent and entirely reversible.

Unlike genetic mutations that cannot be undone, food choices can be changed instantly. Unlike environmental toxins that may persist in the body for years, food effects can begin reversing within days.

The populations that adopted Western foods and developed Western disease rates did not remain sick permanently. In some cases, populations that have moved away from Western processed foods have seen disease rates decline.

More importantly, individuals who have made the shift from processed to whole foods have experienced dramatic health improvements. People with Type 2 diabetes for decades have achieved normal blood glucose. People with heart disease have experienced regression of arterial plaque. People with depression have recovered without medications. People with cognitive decline have recovered mental clarity.[12]

This is not theoretical. This is documented thousands of times over. The human body's capacity to heal when given proper nutrition is extraordinary.

The disconnection from whole foods is not permanent. It is a choice. And it can be reversed through a different choice.

The Path Forward

The modern disconnection from whole foods has created the disease epidemic. Understanding this disconnection is crucial to understanding how to reverse it.

You are not sick because of bad genetics or bad luck or inevitable aging. You are sick because your body is consuming foods it was not designed to consume. Your mitochondria are being poisoned by refined carbohydrates, oxidized seed oils, and processed additives. Your energy production is being disrupted.

But this disruption is reversible.

The solution is not new medications or more sophisticated disease management. The solution is reconnection. Reconnection with the foods humans evolved to consume. Reconnection with whole plants in their natural form. Reconnection with the nutritional patterns that kept humans healthy for hundreds of thousands of years.

This reconnection requires stepping away from the modern food system. It requires stepping away from the convenient, marketed, industrialized food that surrounds you. It requires making different choices.

But these choices are available to you right now. At this moment. You can choose to eat whole plant food. You can choose not to eat processed food. These choices, made repeatedly, accumulate to restore your energy and your health.

The disconnection is real. The damage is documented. But so is the possibility of reconnection.

The next chapter will reveal the unified framework that explains why reconnection works for all diseases. But first, understand that the modern disconnection from whole foods is the root cause of the modern disease epidemic. And reconnection is the path to recovery.

3

THE HEALING FRAMEWORK

The Unified Diagnosis

Here is a truth that will revolutionize how you understand health and disease: Every chronic disease has the same root cause. Not similar causes. Not related causes. The same cause.

Type 2 diabetes, heart disease, Alzheimer's disease, depression, obesity, autoimmune disease, chronic pain these are not separate diseases caused by separate problems. These are different expressions of the same underlying dysfunction: energy system failure.

The names we give these diseases, the diagnostic labels, and the specialized medical terminology obscure this fundamental unity. We treat them as distinct problems requiring different specialists, different medications, different approaches. A person with diabetes sees an endocrinologist. A person with heart disease sees a cardiologist. A person with depression sees a psychiatrist.

But what if this entire framework is wrong?

What if we have been naming symptoms instead of identifying the disease? What if we have been organizing medicine around the organs that fail rather than around the system that is failing?

Consider that a cardiologist treats the heart. An endocrinologist treats the pancreas. A neurologist treats the brain. But what if the problem is not in these organs specifically? What if the problem is in the energy-producing system that all these organs depend on?

When you restore energy production to the heart, the heart functions properly. When you restore energy production to the pancreas, it produces appropriate insulin. When you restore energy production to the brain, it produces appropriate neurotransmitters and maintains appropriate connections.

One intervention. One root cause. Multiple diseases reversed.

This is the healing framework. This is the revolution.

Why Disease Names Are Misleading

Medicine has trained us to think in terms of disease names. We have Type 2 diabetes, heart disease, depression, arthritis, each a distinct entity requiring distinct treatment.

But these names are misleading. They describe organ dysfunction, not the underlying problem.

Consider Type 2 diabetes. The diagnostic label tells you the pancreas is not producing enough insulin, or cells are not responding to insulin, or both. The pancreas is failing. The name describes what the pancreas is doing wrong.

But the pancreas is not inherently broken. The pancreas is energy starved.

The pancreatic beta cells that produce insulin require enormous ATP. When you consume refined carbohydrates, blood glucose spikes repeatedly. The pancreas must respond with massive insulin secretion repeatedly. This constant demand depletes the energy available to the beta cells. They are exhausted. They can no longer produce adequate insulin.

The problem is not the pancreas. The problem is energy insufficiency in the pancreas.

Fix the energy, and the pancreas functions normally again.

Consider heart disease. The diagnostic label tells you arteries are narrowed, atherosclerotic plaque has accumulated, blood flow is restricted. The heart is failing. The name describes what the heart and arteries are doing wrong.

But the arteries are not inherently defective. The arterial endothelium, the inner lining of arteries, is energy starved.

The endothelial cells that line your arteries require ATP to maintain the smooth surface that prevents clot formation, to produce nitric oxide that keeps arteries relaxed, to repair damage, and to maintain the barrier that keeps harmful substances out of artery walls. When these cells become energy starved, they malfunction. They allow oxidized cholesterol and inflammatory compounds to accumulate. Plaque forms. Atherosclerosis develops.

The problem is not the heart or arteries. The problem is energy insufficiency in the cells that maintain arterial health.

Fix the energy, and the arteries function normally again.

Consider depression. The diagnostic label tells you neurotransmitters are imbalanced, particularly serotonin. The brain is malfunctioning. The name describes what brain chemistry is doing wrong.

But the brain is not inherently broken. Specific brain regions are energy starved.

The neurons in brain regions involved in mood regulation particularly the prefrontal cortex, the hippocampus, and the amygdala require enormous amounts of ATP. They maintain thousands of synaptic connections. They produce and recycle neurotransmitters constantly. When energy becomes insufficient, these neurons cannot maintain these connections and cannot produce adequate neurotransmitters.

The problem is not neurotransmitter deficiency primarily. The problem is energy insufficiency in neurons.

Fix the energy, and neurotransmitter production normalizes, connections are maintained, and mood recovers.

This pattern repeats across every chronic disease. We name them based on which organ fails first or most obviously. But the underlying problem in every case is the same: insufficient ATP production.

The diseases are different expressions of one problem: energy dysfunction.

The Organ Vulnerability Hierarchy: Why You Get What You Get

If all chronic diseases share the same root cause of energy insufficiency, why do different people develop different diseases?

The answer lies in the concept of organ vulnerability.

Different organs have different energy demands. Different people have different genetic vulnerabilities, different stress levels, and different organ systems that are already compromised.

When energy becomes insufficient, organs fail in a predictable hierarchy based on their energy demands and vulnerabilities.

THE BRAIN: FIRST TO SHOW SUBTLE DYSFUNCTION

The brain uses approximately 20 percent of the body's total energy at rest. It is extraordinarily energy hungry. When systemic energy decreases, the brain often shows the first subtle signs of brain fog, difficulty concentrating, mood changes, reduced motivation, sleep disturbance.

This is why many people with energy insufficiency first notice cognitive or mood changes before they notice physical symptoms. The brain is the first to be energy rationed.

THE HEART: DEMANDS CONSISTENT, RELENTLESS ENERGY

The heart beats roughly one hundred thousand times daily. It never rests. Each beat requires ATP. The heart uses approximately 25 percent of the body's energy at rest second only to the brain.

When energy becomes insufficient, the heart struggles. Arrhythmias develop (irregular heartbeats caused by energy-starved cardiac cells). Heart function declines. In people whose primary vulnerability is cardiovascular, heart disease becomes the expression of energy insufficiency.

THE PANCREAS: ENERGY DEPLETED BY GLUCOSE SPIKES

The pancreatic beta cells that produce insulin are extraordinarily energy intensive. They must respond to every blood glucose elevation with precisely calibrated insulin secretion. In people eating refined carbohydrates, they are under constant, relentless energy demand.

For people with this vulnerability, those whose pancreas is their weakest link, Type 2 diabetes becomes the expression of energy insufficiency.

THE GUT BARRIER: CRUMBLES WHEN ENERGY STARVED

The intestinal epithelial cells that form the gut barrier require constant ATP to maintain tight junctions between cells. When energy becomes insufficient, these junctions fail. The gut becomes permeable. Bacterial lipopolysaccharides leak through. Systemic inflammation escalates.

For people whose primary vulnerability is digestive, chronic digestive dysfunction, food sensitivities, and gut dysbiosis become their primary expression of energy insufficiency.

THE IMMUNE SYSTEM: BECOMES DYSFUNCTIONAL

Immune cells require enormous ATP to create antibodies, kill pathogens, and maintain immune regulation. When energy becomes insufficient, immune function declines.

For people whose primary vulnerability is immune system, frequent infections or autoimmune dysfunction becomes their expression of energy insufficiency.

THE JOINTS AND CONNECTIVE TISSUE: DETERIORATE

Chondrocytes (cartilage cells) and other joint structures require constant ATP to maintain structural integrity. When energy becomes insufficient, joint cells deteriorate. Inflammation increases. Arthritis develops.

For people whose primary vulnerability is musculoskeletal, arthritis becomes their expression of energy insufficiency.

THE BRAIN AGAIN: ADVANCED DYSFUNCTION

If energy insufficiency progresses long enough without intervention, brain dysfunction becomes severe. Cognitive decline accelerates. Memory loss becomes obvious. Alzheimer's disease and other dementias develop.

THE PATTERN

The pattern is consistent: when energy becomes insufficient, organs fail in order of their energy demands and individual vulnerabilities.

A person with a family history of heart disease and high energy demands on their cardiovascular system may develop heart disease at fifty.

A person with high insulin demand (eating refined carbohydrates constantly) and pancreatic vulnerability may develop diabetes at forty-five.

A person with genetic brain vulnerabilities and poor brain energy metabolism may develop cognitive decline at fifty-five.

A person with multiple vulnerabilities and severe energy insufficiency may develop multiple diseases: diabetes, heart disease, arthritis, and cognitive decline all at once.

But the underlying mechanism in every case is insufficient ATP production.

This is the crucial insight: one root cause, multiple organ manifestations, different organ failure patterns depending on individual vulnerabilities.

The Energy Restoration Framework: One Solution, Multiple Diseases Reversed

Here is where the framework becomes truly revolutionary. When you restore ATP production through reconnection with whole plant foods, every organ that was energy starved begins to recover simultaneously.

You do not need separate treatments for each disease. You do not need diabetes medication for the pancreas, heart medication for the heart, antidepressants for the brain, and arthritis medication for the joints.

You restore energy. The energy-starved organs recover. All the diseases improve together.

This is why the same protocol reverses Type 2 diabetes, heart disease, depression, obesity, arthritis, and cognitive decline. Not because of some mysterious universal compound, but because you are addressing the root cause of energy insufficiency that all these diseases share.

THE SIMULTANEOUS REVERSAL PATTERN

When people adopt whole plant-based nutrition and restore their mitochondrial function, a predictable pattern of improvement occurs:

Days 1–3: Energy-dependent symptoms improve first. Fatigue begins lifting. Mental clarity improves slightly. This is because ATP production begins increasing within days of eliminating refined carbohydrates and inflammatory foods.

Weeks 1–2: Metabolic markers improve. Fasting blood glucose drops. Insulin levels decrease. Weight loss begins (partly water loss as refined carbohydrates and salt are eliminated, partly fat loss as energy becomes available for mobilization).

Weeks 3–4: Physical symptoms improve. Pain and inflammation begin decreasing. Blood pressure begins normalizing. Digestion improves. Sleep quality improves.

Months 2–3: More dramatic improvements. Blood glucose normalizes completely for many. Blood pressure normalizes. Cholesterol and triglycerides improve. Weight loss continues. Mental clarity reaches new levels. Mood stabilizes. Energy becomes abundant.

Months 3–6: Complete reversal is often achieved for many people. Laboratory markers normalize. Medications become unnecessary. Symptoms that seemed permanent resolve completely.

THE UNITY OF MECHANISM EXPLAINS THIS PATTERN

Why do all these improvements happen together?

Because you are restoring energy to all tissues simultaneously. Every organ that was energy starved begins recovering.

The pancreas recovers, so insulin production normalizes diabetes reverses. The heart recovers, so cardiac function improves and heart disease reverses. The brain recovers, so neurotransmitter production normalizes depression reverses. The joints recover, so inflammation decreases and arthritis improves. The gut recovers, so barrier function is restored and digestive health returns. The immune system recovers, so infection resistance improves and health is restored.

This simultaneous improvement is not coincidence. It is the inevitable consequence of restoring the fundamental system energy production that all organs depend on.

WHY THIS EXPLAINS PHENOMENA THAT SEEM PARADOXICAL

From a disease-specific framework, simultaneous improvement seems paradoxical. How can one intervention treat diabetes, heart disease, and depression? These are different diseases caused by different problems.

But from an energy framework, simultaneous improvement is expected. You are addressing the root problem, so of course, multiple diseases improve.

From a disease-specific framework, rapid improvement seems suspicious. Diseases take time to develop; shouldn't they take time to reverse?

But from an energy framework, rapid improvement is expected. Mitochondria can increase ATP production within days of eliminating poisons and providing proper nutrients. Improvement follows naturally.

From a disease-specific framework, medications failing to prevent disease progression seems like a failure of the specific medication. Maybe stronger medication is needed.

But from an energy framework, medication failure is expected. You are not treating the root cause. You are treating symptoms while the root cause of energy insufficiency continues. Of course, disease progresses despite medication.

Every paradox resolves when you understand the unified framework.

The Nature-Based Solution: IN NATURE WE TRUST

This framework is not new. It is not a modern invention. It is a return to the fundamental principle that has guided human health for hundreds of thousands of years.

Your body is designed to consume and thrive on whole plant foods. This is not an opinion. This is fact based on evolutionary design.

Your digestive system is designed for plants. Your teeth are designed to grind fibrous plant material. Your gut microbiome evolved to ferment plant fiber. Your metabolic pathways are optimized for plant-based nutrition.

Your mitochondria evolved their energy-producing machinery on the fuel that plants provide.

This is not about ideology or philosophy. This is about biological design.

Nature designed you to consume plants. Nature designed plants to nourish you. The two are perfectly matched the result of millions of years of coevolution.

When you consume what nature designed you to consume, your body functions optimally. Your energy production is optimal. Your health is optimal.

When you consume what nature did not design you to consume refined carbohydrates, oxidized seed oils, processed additives your body malfunctions. Your energy production declines. Your health deteriorates.

This is the framework:

IN NATURE WE TRUST.

Not in pharmaceutical medications designed in laboratories to mask symptoms. Not in processed foods designed in factories to maximize profit and encourage overeating. Not in medical recommendations shaped by industries with financial incentives to perpetuate disease.

Trust in nature. Trust in the foods your ancestors ate for hundreds of thousands of years. Trust in the biological design that evolution created.

When you align with nature when you consume the foods nature designed you to consume your body heals naturally. Your mitochondria function optimally. Your energy is abundant. Your health is restored.

This is not faith. This is biology.

The Reversal Is Predictable and Reliable

One of the most powerful aspects of understanding the energy framework is that the reversal is predictable.

When you restore ATP production through whole plant-based nutrition, healing follows naturally. It is not mysterious. It is not magical. It is a biological inevitability.

Energy-starved cells recover when given energy and the nutrients required to produce it. This is not controversial. This is basic biochemistry.

The predictability means you can anticipate what will happen. You can have confidence that if you follow the protocol if you restore your energy production your body will heal.

This is radically different from conventional medicine's uncertainty. A person taking medication does not know if it will work. The medication might help. It might not. Side effects are unpredictable. Disease progression is unpredictable.

But with energy restoration through whole plant nutrition, the outcome is remarkably predictable. Blood glucose normalizes within weeks. Blood pressure normalizes within weeks. Weight normalizes within months. Symptoms resolve. Disease reverses.

This predictability is not because every person is identical. Individual variation in timeline and magnitude is real. But the direction of change is consistent: energy restoration leads to health restoration.

Symptoms Are Messages, Not Problems

Understanding the energy framework changes how you relate to your symptoms.

Symptoms are not the problem. Symptoms are messages. Your body's way of telling you that energy is insufficient.

Fatigue is the message that your cells do not have adequate ATP. Brain fog is the message that your brain is energy rationed. High blood pressure is the message that your blood vessels cannot relax because energy is insufficient. Elevated blood glucose is the message that your pancreas cannot produce adequate insulin because energy is insufficient. Depression is the message that your brain is energy starved in regions that regulate mood. Pain and inflammation are the message that tissues are damaged and energy is insufficient for repair.

When you suppress these messages with medications, you silence the alarm without addressing the fire.

But when you understand these messages and address the underlying energy insufficiency, the messages naturally resolve because the problem is solved.

A person takes blood pressure medication, and their blood pressure number goes down. They think they are healthy. But their vessels are still dysfunctional; the medication is just forcing them into a lower pressure state.

A person restores their energy production, and their blood pressure normalizes because their vessels actually recover function. They are genuinely healthy, not just symptomatically managed.

The difference is profound.

Why Medications Often Fail to Prevent Disease Progression

This explains a phenomenon that conventional medicine struggles to explain: Why do patients on medications for chronic diseases often experience continued disease progression?

A person takes blood pressure medication, and their pressure is controlled, but within a few years, their kidneys begin to fail anyway.

A person takes cholesterol medication and their cholesterol is lowered, but they still have a heart attack.

A person takes diabetes medication and their glucose is controlled, but they still develop diabetic complications.

From a disease-specific framework, this seems like medication failure. Maybe stronger medication is needed.

But from an energy framework, this progression is expected. You are controlling a symptom while the root cause continues. The body is still energy starved. Tissues are still being damaged by insufficient ATP. The disease progresses because you have not addressed the reason it started.

It is like treating fever with ice while the infection continues spreading. The fever is suppressed, but the patient still gets sicker because the underlying problem of the infection is not addressed.

When you address the root cause of energy insufficiency the disease stops progressing and reverses.

The Framework Predicts Observable Outcomes

The most powerful test of a scientific framework is whether it predicts observable outcomes.

The energy framework predicts:

- Energy-starved organs will show dysfunction corresponding to their vulnerability.
- Restoring energy production will improve all organs simultaneously.
- Rapid improvement will occur within days to weeks.
- Laboratory markers will normalize within weeks to months.

- Disease reversal will be documented within months.
- Long-term improvements will be sustained as long as energy production remains optimal.

All of these predictions are confirmed by thousands of documented cases. The framework predicts and reality confirms.

In contrast, the disease-specific framework predicts:

- Different diseases require different treatments.
- Multiple diseases require multiple medications.
- Disease progression is inevitable despite treatment.
- Management is the goal, not reversal.

These predictions are contradicted by what happens when people restore their energy production. All diseases improve together. Multiple medications become unnecessary. Disease reverses, not just progresses more slowly.

The energy framework is not just more elegant. It is more predictive. It is more aligned with what actually happens.

The Unity Makes Sense Evolutionarily

From an evolutionary perspective, the energy framework makes perfect sense.

Humans evolved over millions of years in environments where food, plant foods were the primary variable affecting survival. Starvation was a constant threat. Natural selection favored bodies that could thrive on available plant foods and that responded to nutritional sufficiency with health and to nutritional insufficiency with disease signals.

This is not complicated. This is elegant.

Your body did not evolve separate systems for regulating blood glucose, blood pressure, mood, digestion, immunity, and all other functions. Your body evolved one fundamental system: the energy-producing system.

All other systems, all organ systems depend on this fundamental energy system.

When energy is abundant, all systems function optimally. When energy is scarce, all systems show signs of dysfunction proportional to their individual vulnerabilities.

This is not new medicine. This is old medicine based on evolutionary biology.

The Path to Health Is Clear

Understanding the healing framework clarifies the path to health.

You do not need to treat your diabetes and your heart disease and your depression separately. You do not need multiple specialists and multiple medications and multiple treatment plans.

You need to address one thing: your energy production.

Restore your energy production, and your body heals. All the diseases that were expressions of energy insufficiency improve simultaneously.

The path is clear:

1. Understand that all your chronic diseases share a root cause of energy insufficiency.
2. Understand that energy insufficiency is caused by consuming foods your body was not designed to consume.
3. Understand that energy sufficiency is restored by consuming foods your body evolved to consume.
4. Make the choice to reconnect with whole plant foods.
5. Trust your body's healing capacity.
6. Watch as your health is restored.

This is not complicated medicine. This is elegant biology.

This is the healing framework.

4

IN NATURE WE TRUST: PHILOSOPHY AND SCIENCE

A Radical Proposition

In this moment, in this culture, what I am about to propose is radical.

Trust nature more than you trust medicine. Trust the foods nature provides more than you trust pharmaceutical medications. Trust your body's healing capacity more than you trust disease management protocols. Trust evolution's wisdom more than you trust industry's promises.

This is radical because modern culture has trained you to distrust nature and trust human technology. Nature is presented as chaotic, dangerous, and inferior. Technology is presented as orderly, safe, and superior.

We have been taught that nature is something to be conquered, controlled, and improved upon. We have been taught that human ingenuity in the form of medicine, technology, and industry is our salvation.

We have been trained to ask: Can modern medicine cure this disease? Can pharmaceutical companies solve this problem? Can food corporations provide adequate nutrition?

The answer conventional culture gives is yes, trust human technology. Nature is insufficient.

But what if this is wrong?

What if nature is not inferior? What if nature's solutions are superior to human creations? What if the problem is not that nature is insufficient, but that we have abandoned nature and adopted inferior substitutes?

What if trusting nature is not primitive faith but sophisticated science?

The Nature vs. Technology False Dichotomy

Modern culture presents a false choice: nature or technology. You must choose one or the other.

This is wrong.

The dichotomy itself is the problem.

In reality, the most advanced science is not trying to replace nature. The most advanced science is trying to understand nature and align with it.

Modern medicine's greatest successes come when it works with nature, not against it. Vaccines work by training the immune system with nature's own defense mechanism. Antibiotics work by harnessing natural compounds produced by microorganisms. Surgery works by assisting the body's own healing mechanisms.

Modern medicine's greatest failures come when it tries to replace nature with artificial substitutes.

Medications that attempt to artificially modify neurotransmitter levels instead of addressing why neurotransmitter production is insufficient often fail and create dependence.

Dietary recommendations that attempt to replace nature's foods with processed substitutes create disease instead of health.

Pharmaceutical interventions that attempt to artificially lower blood pressure instead of healing the vascular system that naturally regulates blood pressure fail to prevent disease progression.

The problem is not technology itself. The problem is technology that tries to replace nature rather than align with it.

The right approach is to trust nature's design. Use technology to understand it. Use technology to support alignment with it. But do not use technology to replace it.

This is what IN NATURE WE TRUST means.

Not antitechnology. Not antimedicine. But pro-alignment with nature. Pro-understanding how nature works. Pro-using technology in service of working with nature, not against it.

The Coevolution: Humans and Plants

To understand why trusting nature is scientifically justified, you must understand the extraordinary coevolution that created the human body and plant foods.

Humans did not evolve in isolation. Humans evolved in ecosystems filled with plants. For millions of years, as humans evolved, plants were evolving alongside us.

Plants developed and compounds phytonutrients as chemical defenses. These compounds protected plants from insects, pathogens, and damage.

Humans, consuming these plants, were exposed to these phytonutrients. Over millions of years, human bodies adapted to these compounds. Our bodies learned to recognize them. Our bodies developed ways to use them for our own health.

This is not a coincidence. This is coevolution.

For example, berries contain anthocyanins polyphenols that give berries their color and serve as the plant's defense against insects. Humans consuming berries became exposed to anthocyanins. Over millions of years, human brains developed ways to use anthocyanins to enhance mitochondrial function and improve cognitive ability.

Today, berries are among the most brain-healthy foods available. Not because humans engineered berries to be brain healthy. But because berries and humans coevolved together. The plant's defense compounds became human health-promoting compounds.

This pattern repeats throughout the plant kingdom. Thousands of plant compounds that evolved as plant defenses have become human health-promoting compounds.

This is not an accident. This is the result of millions of years of coevolution.

Nature has spent millions of years optimizing the relationship between human bodies and plant foods. No human researcher, no matter how intelligent or well-resourced, could design a food system as sophisticated as what nature has created.

Consider the nutritional package of a single apple:

- Carbohydrates for energy
- Fiber for gut health and glucose modulation
- Polyphenols for antioxidant and anti-inflammatory benefit
- Vitamins and minerals as cofactors in energy production
- Water for hydration
- Natural compounds that signal to your genes that food is abundant

An apple is not just nutrition. An apple is an information package. The compounds in the apple signal to your body, "Nutritious food is available. Heal. Thrive. Reproduce." Your body responds to this information by activating healing pathways.

A processed food providing the same calories and macronutrients cannot replicate this. The processed food provides energy, but it does not provide the signal. Your body does not receive the message that nutritious food is available. Instead, it receives signals of nutritional insufficiency and responds by initiating stress responses.

This is the difference between nature and human substitutes. Nature provides not just nutrition, but information. Human creations provide calories, but often misinformation.

The Evolutionary Argument:
Why Nature's Design Is Superior

From an evolutionary perspective, trusting nature is not faith. It is science.

Your body was shaped by millions of years of natural selection. Every aspect of your physiology was selected because it promoted survival and reproduction in ancestral environments.

Your digestive system evolved in environments where food was whole plants. Your gut microbiome evolved to ferment plant fiber. Your metabolic pathways evolved to process plant-based nutrition. Your mitochondria evolved to generate ATP from plant fuels.

This evolution created a body perfectly designed to consume and thrive on whole plants.

Now contrast this with human-created foods. Refined carbohydrates have existed for 150 years. Industrial seed oils have existed for one hundred years. Ultra-processed foods have existed for fifty years. Artificial sweeteners have existed for seventy years.

Your body has had zero evolutionary time to adapt to these fake foods. These foods are evolutionarily novel. Your body has no evolutionary preparation for them.

When you consume evolutionarily novel foods, your body responds as though it is being poisoned. Because, in a sense, it is. These foods are not compatible with your evolved physiology.

This is why processed foods cause disease. Not because they contain bad ingredients, but because they are fundamentally incompatible with the body they are being consumed by.

In contrast, whole plant foods are evolutionarily ancient. Your body spent hundreds of thousands of years evolving to consume them. Your body knows exactly what to do with them. Your physiology responds with health and vitality.

From an evolutionary perspective, the choice is clear: Consume what your body evolved to consume. Reject what your body has never encountered.

This is not ideology. This is applied evolutionary biology.

The Scientific Validation:
Nature's Superiority Is Measurable

The philosophical and evolutionary arguments for trusting nature are strong. But the scientific argument is strongest.

Modern science can measure what happens when humans consume nature's foods versus human-created substitutes.

THE BLOOD SUGAR RESPONSE

When you consume a whole apple, your blood glucose rises gradually. The fiber in the apple slows glucose absorption. The whole food provides a sustained, moderate glucose elevation.

Your pancreas responds with appropriate insulin secretion. Your cells accept the glucose. Your mitochondria process it efficiently. Your energy is sustained.

When you consume refined carbohydrates providing the same amount of glucose, your blood glucose spikes dramatically. Glucose floods the bloodstream within minutes.[1,2]

Your pancreas responds with excessive insulin secretion. Your cells are overwhelmed. Excess glucose is converted to fat. Your mitochondria are damaged by the free radicals generated during this excess. Your energy crashes afterward.

Measurement shows these differences in real time with continuous glucose monitors. Nature's food equals stable glucose. Human substitute equals chaotic glucose spikes.

THE MICROBIOME RESPONSE

When you consume whole plant foods high in fiber, your gut microbiome flourishes. Beneficial bacteria proliferate. Short-chain fatty acid production increases. Inflammatory markers decrease.

When you consume processed foods lacking fiber and containing additives, your gut microbiome suffers. Beneficial bacteria die. Harmful bacteria proliferate. Inflammatory markers increase. The gut barrier deteriorates.

Measurement through microbiome analysis shows these differences clearly. Nature's food provides a thriving microbiome while human food substitutes provide dysbiosis and inflammation.

THE MITOCHONDRIAL RESPONSE

When you consume whole plant foods rich in polyphenols and minerals, your mitochondria thrive. Mitochondrial density increases. ATP production increases. Free radical production decreases.

When you consume processed foods lacking polyphenols and minerals and containing oxidized seed oils, your mitochondria deteriorate. Mitochondrial density decreases. ATP production decreases. Free radical production increases.

Measurement through cellular studies shows these differences. Nature's food provides a thriving mitochondria while human substitutes provide dysfunctional mitochondria.

THE INFLAMMATORY RESPONSE

When you consume whole plant foods, systemic inflammation decreases. Inflammatory markers (C-reactive protein, IL-6, TNF-alpha) decline. Immune dysregulation resolves.

When you consume processed foods, particularly those with additives and emulsifiers, systemic inflammation increases. Inflammatory markers rise. Immune dysregulation worsens.

Measurement shows these differences in laboratory markers. Nature's food reduces inflammation while human food substitutes increase inflammation.

THE REAL-WORLD CLINICAL OUTCOMES

When populations consume whole plant-based diets, chronic disease rates are near zero.

When populations consume processed food diets, chronic disease rates are epidemic.

When individuals switch from processed to whole plant-based diets, disease reversal occurs within weeks to months.

The science is consistent and overwhelming: nature's foods produce measurably superior health outcomes compared to human-created substitutes.

WHAT NATURE HAS SOLVED: FOUR BILLION YEARS OF R&D

Here is a perspective that should humble anyone who believes human technology is superior to nature: Nature has been conducting research and development for four billion years.

Four billion years of evolution. Four billion years of trial and error. Four billion years of optimization.

The result is life on Earth. An astonishing diversity of organisms, all perfectly adapted to their environments, all with physiology optimized for survival and thriving.

Humans have been conducting research for perhaps two hundred years in the modern scientific era. We have been trying to improve upon what nature created through technology.

We are children trying to improve upon a masterpiece created by a genius with four billion years of experience.

This is not to say human research and technology are worthless. Human research has revealed how nature works. Human technology has created many beneficial things. But the idea that human technology is superior to nature's solutions in areas like nutrition and health is arrogance.

Nature has solved the problem of health. It has solved how to create foods that nourish human bodies optimally. It has solved how to create the nutrients and compounds needed for thriving.

The problem is not that nature's solutions are insufficient. The problem is that we have abandoned nature's solutions and tried to replace them with inferior human creations.

Returning to nature's solutions is not regression. It is wisdom.

THE CORPORATE CAPTURE: HOW WE WERE TRAINED TO DISTRUST NATURE

If nature's solutions are so superior, why has modern culture adopted processed foods?

The answer lies in corporate capture of science, medicine, and public perception.

Food corporations discovered that processed foods are more profitable than whole foods. Whole foods are perishable, require refrigeration, have low profit margins, and require minimal corporate infrastructure. Processed foods last indefinitely, require no refrigeration, have high profit margins, and can only be manufactured by large corporations.

So food corporations invested billions in marketing, in influencing science, and in shaping public perception to convince people that processed foods were modern, convenient, and desirable.

Pharmaceutical corporations discovered that treating diseases with medications is more profitable than preventing disease through nutrition. A person on a statin for heart disease generates thousands of dollars in profit annually. A person who prevents heart disease through diet generates zero profit.

So pharmaceutical corporations invested billions in marketing medications, in funding medical research that emphasizes pharmaceutical solutions, and in shaping medical education to focus on drugs rather than nutrition.

The result is a coordinated effort, not usually through explicit conspiracy but through aligned financial incentives, to train the population to distrust nature and trust corporate products instead.

We were trained to believe:

- Nature's foods are inefficient and insufficient.
- Processed foods are modern and progress.
- Medications are the solution to disease.
- Doctors are authorities on health.

But what if these beliefs are wrong? What if they were deliberately cultivated to serve corporate interests?

What if the truth is:

- Nature's foods are perfectly designed for human health.
- Processed foods are poisons created for profit.
- Medications often manage symptoms while disease continues.
- True health requires alignment with nature, not corporate products.

The training we received was thorough and effective. Most people believe the false narrative. But the narrative is false.

The truth is simpler and more empowering: trust nature. Consume what nature designed you to consume. Your body will heal.

THE RADICAL ACT: CHOOSING NATURE OVER CORPORATE SUBSTITUTES

In modern culture, choosing to trust nature is a radical act.

It means rejecting marketing messages that surround you constantly. It means making different choices than what the mainstream promotes. It means being willing to be different, to be outside the cultural norm.

It means walking past the processed food aisles and buying vegetables. It means preparing meals from scratch instead of buying convenience foods. It means investing time in cooking and eating real food when processed foods are faster.

It means questioning medical recommendations shaped by industry. It means asking: Is this recommendation based on what serves my health, or on what serves corporate profits?

It means trusting your own body's signals instead of trusting authorities who may be compromised by industry influence.

This is not easy. Culture and marketing push relentlessly toward processed foods and pharmaceutical solutions. Family members may question your choices. Friends may think you are extreme.

But this radical act of choosing nature is the most powerful choice you can make for your health.

Because when you choose nature, you choose to align yourself with four billion years of optimization. You choose to trust a system vastly more sophisticated and wiser than any human creation.

THE PERMISSION: YOU ARE ALLOWED TO TRUST NATURE

Here is something no one tells you: You are allowed to trust nature more than you trust the recommendations of authorities compromised by industry. You are allowed to question medical advice shaped by pharmaceutical industry funding. You are allowed to reject processed foods marketed as healthy.

You are allowed to make different choices. You are allowed to be outside the mainstream. You are allowed to trust your own body's wisdom.

Your body knows what it needs. It evolved in alignment with nature for millions of years. It knows how to use whole plant foods for health. It knows how to heal when given proper nutrition.

The only question is will you listen to your body, or will you continue listening to marketing messages and industry-influenced recommendations?

The choice is yours. But know this, the choice has consequences.

Choose processed foods and industry-influenced medicine, and your body will progressively deteriorate. Disease will develop. You will become dependent on medications. Your health will decline.

Choose nature. Choose whole plants. Choose to align with your evolutionary design. And your body will thrive. Energy will become abundant. Disease will reverse. Health will be restored.

The choice is real. The consequences are real. The outcome is your choice.

IN NATURE WE TRUST: THE OPERATING PRINCIPLE

This, then, is what IN NATURE WE TRUST means:

We trust that nature has designed foods perfectly suited to human physiology. We trust that four billion years of evolution has created plant foods optimally composed to nourish human bodies. We trust that no human creation can improve upon this design.

We trust that nature's solutions are superior to human-created substitutes. We trust that whole foods will produce better health outcomes than processed foods. We trust that alignment with evolutionary design produces health. We trust that disease is the body's signal that we are not aligned with our evolutionary design.

We trust that the human body possesses extraordinary healing capacity. We trust that given proper nutrition the foods we evolved to consume the body will heal itself. We trust that symptoms will resolve, disease will reverse, and health will be restored.

We trust that corporate profit motives have corrupted our understanding of health. We trust that the food and pharmaceutical industries have deliberately shaped science, medicine, and public perception to serve profit rather than health. We trust that these interests have compromised conventional recommendations.

We trust that individual choice can override cultural training. We trust that each person can make the choice to reconnect with nature, despite the marketing and cultural pressure to consume processed foods and medications. We trust that this choice, made daily, accumulates to restore health.

We trust that this alignment with nature is not regression but progression. We trust that returning to foods humans evolved to consume is not primitive but wise. We trust that this is not abandoning modern benefits but reclaiming evolutionary wisdom while maintaining the genuine benefits of modern medicine and technology.

This is IN NATURE WE TRUST.

Not blind faith. Not antitechnology. Not antimedicine.

But clear-eyed recognition that in the domain of nutrition and chronic disease, nature's solutions are superior to human creations. Recognition that four billion years of evolution has created sophistication that human technology has not yet matched. Recognition that the primary cause of the chronic disease epidemic is disconnection from the foods we evolved to consume. Recognition that the primary solution is reconnection with nature.

The Integration: Using Modern Tools to Align with Nature

Trusting nature does not mean rejecting all modern tools and knowledge.

Modern medicine has genuine value. Antibiotics for serious infections. Surgery for acute injuries. Emergency medicine for acute crises. These are legitimate uses of modern medical technology.

Modern science has genuine value. Understanding how nutrients work. Understanding how mitochondria function. Understanding the mechanisms by which foods affect health. This knowledge comes from modern science and is valuable.

Modern monitoring tools have genuine value. Glucose monitors for tracking blood glucose improvement. Blood tests for measuring health markers. These tools can provide valuable feedback.

The distinction is this:

Use modern tools to understand and support alignment with nature. Do not use modern tools to replace or override nature.

Use blood tests to verify that your health markers are improving as you align with whole plant foods. Use continuous glucose monitors to see how different whole foods affect your glucose. Use modern medicine when acute crises require intervention.

But do not use pharmaceuticals to replace the healing that comes from restoring energy production through proper nutrition. Do not use processed foods to replace whole foods. Do not rely on industry recommendations to guide your choices when those recommendations are compromised by profit motives.

The path forward integrates the best of both; nature's wisdom about nutrition and health, combined with modern tools to support and verify alignment with that wisdom.

The Revolutionary Implication

Here is what becomes clear when you truly understand IN NATURE WE TRUST: You do not need the medical establishment to be healthy.

You do not need doctors' permission. You do not need pharmaceutical medications. You do not need expensive interventions or procedures.

What you need is food. Whole plant foods. The raw foods nature designed for you.

That is it. That is the entire solution.

This is revolutionary because it removes the medical establishment's power over your health. You are not dependent on their expertise. You are not dependent on their medications. You are not dependent on their recommendations.

You are dependent only on your access to whole plant foods and your willingness to consume them.

This shift in power from external authorities to your own choice and your own body's wisdom is the deepest revolution available.

You can reclaim your health. You can reverse disease. You can achieve vitality and energy and life that exceeds what you thought possible.

Not through doctors' permission. Not through medications. Not through medical procedures.

Through simple reconnection with the foods your body evolved to consume.

This is the revolution. This is what IN NATURE WE TRUST means.

Moving Forward

The next chapter will provide the practical framework for implementing this philosophy. You will learn specifically how to reconnect with nature. You will learn what foods to consume and why. You will learn how to transform your health through alignment with nature's design.

But first, let the profound simplicity of this principle settle into your being: Your body is not broken. Your body is not fundamentally flawed. Your body is not your enemy.

Your body is a masterpiece of four billion years of evolution. Your body is perfectly designed to consume whole plant foods and thrive on them. Your body possesses extraordinary healing capacity.

The only question is will you give your body what it needs?

Will you choose to trust nature? Will you choose to align with your evolutionary design? Will you choose to reconnect with the foods that created you and can heal you?

If you choose yes, if you truly choose to trust nature, everything changes.

Your health changes. Your energy changes. Your life changes.

IN NATURE WE TRUST.

Not because it is easy. But because it works.

Not because it is fashionable. But because it is true.

Not because authorities recommend it. But because your four-billion-year evolutionary history recommends it.

Trust nature. Trust your body. Trust the healing that follows when you align with your evolutionary design.

The path is clear. The choice is yours.

5

THE RAW FOOD PROTOCOL: ENERGY ALIGNMENT OVERVIEW

The Bridge: From Philosophy to Practice

You now understand that life is fundamentally energy. You know that all chronic disease stems from energy system dysfunction. You comprehend that disconnection from natural foods created this dysfunction. You see that reconnection through natural alignment restores this energy.

But understanding is not yet transformation.

This chapter bridges that gap. It introduces the protocol not as a rigid diet to follow, but as a framework for realigning your body's energy systems with what nature designed. It answers the essential question: How do I actually do this?

The answer is simpler than modern nutrition makes it seem. And more profound.

The Viability Principle: Why Living Food Creates Living Energy

There is a principle that distinguishes this protocol from every other dietary approach. It separates genuine health restoration from calorie manipulation. It explains why this protocol works when others fail. It's called the *Viability Principle*.

UNDERSTANDING THE PRINCIPLE

Take a seed in your hand. A raw seed, perhaps a lentil, a grain of wheat, an apple seed. Hold it. Feel its potential.

This seed contains something profound—the biological capacity to generate new life. Plant it in soil, water it, expose it to sunlight, and under the right conditions, something extraordinary happens. That seed becomes a plant. A plant becomes sustenance. Life generates from that small potential.

This capacity reveals something scientifically true about that seed: it is alive. Its enzymatic systems are intact and active. Its polyphenols and phytonutrients are metabolically available. Its mitochondrial-supporting compounds are present in their most bioactive form. Its life force is present not as metaphor, but as measurable biological reality.

Now cook that seed.

Apply heat. Break down cellular structures. Denature proteins. Inactivate enzymes. Damage polyphenols. Eliminate the conditions necessary for biological function.

Now, plant that cooked seed. Water it. Wait.

Nothing happens. It will never grow. Its enzymatic systems are irreversibly damaged. Its capacity for life is extinct. Its life force is gone. It's dead.

You have transformed living material into dead material. You have not created poison; you have created matter. Matter with caloric content, certainly. Matter that can be broken down and processed for energy extraction. But matter that has lost its essential biological vitality.

Your body is a living system.

And here is what conventional nutrition fundamentally misses: living systems don't merely need calories. They need metabolic activation.

The Difference Between Calories and Life Energy

This distinction is everything.

A calorie is a unit of energy measurement. It's a quantifiable amount of heat that can be extracted from food. You can extract calories from almost anything: processed seed oil, refined sugar, chemically modified ingredients. Your digestive system breaks these down, your mitochondria extract ATP, you have fuel.

But fuel and life energy are not synonymous.

CALORIES ARE POTENTIAL ENERGY. LIFE ENERGY IS ACTIVATED POTENTIAL.

When you consume a living food, a raw vegetable, a raw fruit, a raw seed, you're not just ingesting nutrients. You're ingesting a complex, intact biological system. Your digestive enzymes meet their enzymatic counterparts in the food. Your metabolic processes recognize the food's intricate structure. Your mitochondria activate in response to genuine biological signals.

Your body's enzyme systems light up. Your metabolic cascade activates. Your cellular energy production optimizes.

When you consume dead food, processed, refined, cooked at high temperatures, you're ingesting broken-down dead matter. Your digestive system must work harder to extract what remains. Your mitochondria must compensate for missing enzymatic support. Your metabolic activation is suppressed because the biological signals that normally activate it are absent.

You extract calories. But you do not activate life energy.

This is why people on the standard American diet (SAD) high in processed, cooked, refined foods report constant fatigue despite adequate calorie consumption. Their mitochondria are undernourished not in calories, but in metabolic activation signals.

This is why people who transition to living foods report immediate energy surges, often within days, despite similar or even lower calorie consumption. They're not getting more fuel. They're getting activated fuel. Their mitochondria are receiving the biological signals they evolved to recognize. Their enzyme systems are activating optimally.

That's the difference. That's the Viability Principle.

The Viable Seed Test: Your Measuring Stick

This principle gives you an objective, elegant test for any food you consume.

Ask yourself: If I planted this, would it grow?

This simple question reveals everything you need to know about whether food contains life force or dead matter.

Raw apple seed? → Plant it, it grows → Contains life force → Eat it

Cooked apple seed? → Plant it, nothing happens → Life force dead → Don't expect living energy

Raw lentils? → Can sprout under right conditions → Metabolic activation intact → Provides life energy

Cooked lentils? → Cannot sprout, never will → Enzymatic systems deactivated → Provides calories only

White rice (refined)? → Never could grow; embryo removed → Dead material from inception → Minimal living energy

Brown rice (whole)? → Could germinate, life potential present → Still contains biological viability → Better energy potential

Whole wheat grain (raw)? → Can sprout, is alive → Contains full enzymatic systems → Maximum life energy

Whole wheat flour (cooked, baked)? → Cannot sprout, heat destroyed viability → Life force gone → Calories without activation

Raw broccoli? → Alive, enzymes intact, cell structures preserved → Metabolic activation potential high → Genuine life energy

Steamed broccoli (gentle cooking)? → Partially compromised, some enzymes damaged → Reduced but substantial life energy → Still infinitely superior to processed

Broccoli powder (processed)? → Life force largely destroyed → Minimal metabolic activation → Mostly calories, minimal energy

This test is:

Objective—Verifiable, not subjective preference

Memorable—Easy principle to carry into every food decision

Powerful—Makes the point viscerally and practically

Scientifically valid—Germination capacity proves enzymatic and metabolic integrity

Nonjudgmental—Explains rather than condemns

Why Living Systems Thrive on Living Materials

This principle isn't mystical. It's biochemical.

When you eat a living food, you're consuming:

Active Enzymes

Raw foods contain thousands of active enzymatic systems.

These enzymes begin breaking down the food's components immediately upon contact with your saliva.

Your digestive system doesn't have to do all the work alone.

Your pancreas, which produces digestive enzymes, doesn't have to work as hard.

Result: More efficient nutrient extraction with less metabolic effort

Cooked foods? The enzymes are denatured. Your digestive system must compensate by producing more enzymes. Your pancreas must work harder. Your mitochondria must expend more energy on digestion, leaving less available for cellular health and energy production.

Intact Polyphenols

Raw foods contain thousands of intact polyphenol structures.

Polyphenols are the signaling molecules that activate your antioxidant systems.

These polyphenols are recognized by your cells as "this is health" signals.

Your cellular defense systems activate in response.

Result: Optimized inflammation management and cellular repair

Cooked foods? Many polyphenols are damaged or destroyed by heat. The signaling molecules your cells evolved to recognize are gone or distorted. Your cells don't receive the activation signals they evolved to receive.

Intact Cellular Structure

Raw foods contain complete cellular matrices.

Plant cells have cell walls (intact in raw foods).

The fiber structure, nutrient density, and nutrient distribution are all preserved.

Your microbiome recognizes these structures and feeds on them.

Result: Optimal gut health and microbiome vitality

Cooked foods? The cellular walls break down. The structure becomes homogenous. Your microbiome has less diversity to work with. Your gut health suffers.

Metabolic Recognition Signals

Your body evolved to recognize living plant material.

Millions of years of evolution taught your mitochondria "When you encounter intact, living plant material, activate maximally."

Raw foods trigger this ancestral recognition.

Your metabolic systems respond with optimization.

Result: Energy production peaks; vitality surges

Cooked dead foods? The recognition signals are altered or eliminated. Your mitochondria don't receive the "go activate" signal. Your metabolism stays subdued.

What the Protocol Is Not

Before explaining what the protocol is, let's be clear about what it isn't.

It is not a raw food cult.

This protocol is not dogmatic about exclusively raw foods. Legumes and grains cannot be consumed raw, they're indigestible. Some vegetables are more bioavailable when cooked slightly. Some populations have thrived on cooked whole foods for generations.

The protocol is not "raw or nothing." It's "whole and living, raw when possible, gently cooked when necessary."

It is not extreme or restrictive.

This protocol is not about deprivation. You're not counting calories. You're not restricting quantities. You're not banning foods temporarily. The framework is simple: unlimited living foods.

It is not another diet that will fail.

Most diets fail because they work against your body's biology. They restrict energy intake, so your mitochondria adapt by reducing energy production. You get tired. You feel deprived. You quit.

This protocol works *with* your body's biology. It provides the metabolic activation your mitochondria evolved to recognize. Your body wants to do this. Sustainability emerges naturally because your body is getting what it needs.

The Protocol: Simple Framework for Energy Alignment

The protocol can be summarized in a single principle: Maximize living plant foods and minimize everything else (raw first—not perfection).

That's it.

WHAT'S INCLUDED: FOODS THAT PASS THE VIABLE SEED TEST

Raw, living foods (unlimited):

Vegetables—All raw vegetables in unlimited quantities. Sweet potato, avocado, potato, spinach, kale, broccoli, cauliflower, carrots, beets, peppers, cucumbers, tomatoes, mushrooms, and so on. These are the foundations. Maximum enzyme content. Maximum polyphenol activity. Maximum life energy.

Fruits—All raw fruits in unlimited quantities. Berries, apples, oranges, bananas, grapes, melons, and so on. Nature's perfect packages of living carbohydrates, vitamins, minerals, and phytonutrients.

Nuts and seeds—Raw nuts and seeds. Almonds, walnuts, sunflower seeds, pumpkin seeds, chia seeds, flax seeds, hemp seeds. These contain living enzymes and healthy fats in their most bioavailable form.

Sprouted legumes and grains—If you sprout them, they pass the viable seed test. Sprouted lentils, sprouted chickpeas, sprouted grains. Sprouting reactivates enzymatic systems and increases nutrient bioavailability dramatically.

Gently cooked whole foods (regular basis):

Whole legumes—Cooked lentils, beans, chickpeas. The whole legume structure is preserved. Viability is compromised by cooking, but the whole structure remains intact. These provide sustained energy and micronutrient density.

Whole grains—Brown rice, quinoa, millet, oats, barley. Cooked whole, with bran and germ intact. Life potential is reduced by cooking, but biological structure remains. These support sustained energy release.

Lightly cooked vegetables—Steamed or lightly sautéed vegetables. Some enzyme loss, but cellular structure largely preserved. Still vastly superior to raw in some cases (lycopene in cooked tomatoes, for instance).

WHAT'S EXCLUDED: FOODS THAT FAIL THE VIABLE SEED TEST

Never growing:

Refined carbohydrates—White rice, white flour, refined bread. The living embryo and bran are removed. Nothing could ever grow from these. They're dead matter from inception. They provide calories but no life energy. They cause glucose dysregulation and metabolic chaos.

Processed seed oils—Vegetable oil, canola oil, soybean oil. These are extracted through heat and chemicals. The seed cannot grow from oil; it's pure processed extraction. These create oxidative stress and mitochondrial dysfunction.

Processed foods—Anything with extracted, refined, chemically modified, or ultraprocessed components. Packaged foods, fast foods, frozen dinners (with added oils and chemicals). These contain no life force and actively disrupt your energy systems.

Added sugars—Refined sugar, high fructose corn syrup, agave nectar. These are extracted, concentrated calories with no life potential. They spike glucose, dysregulate insulin, and crash mitochondrial function.

Artificial additives—Colors, flavors, preservatives, emulsifiers. These are chemicals your body doesn't recognize. They're not food; they're foreign substances that disrupt your cellular function.

Animal products—While meat and dairy were part of historical diets, plant-based whole foods provide the same or superior energy with less inflammatory burden. For energy optimization, plant-based is superior.

Why Each Element Matters: The Energy Perspective

WHY WHOLE FOODS?

Processing separates components. Separation destroys the synergy.

A whole food is a symphony of components working together: fiber, polyphenols, vitamins, minerals, enzymes, cell wall structures. When the components work together in their natural configuration, they activate complex metabolic cascades.

Extracted components are isolated instruments playing alone.

Processing removes the fiber, oxidizes the polyphenols, damages the enzymes, and disrupts the cellular matrix. What remains is nutritionally quantifiable but energetically inert.

Whole foods activate your energy systems. Processed components don't.

WHY PLANT-BASED?

Evolution chose plants as humans' primary fuel.

Your digestive system is optimized for plant foods. Your teeth structure, your stomach acid, your intestinal length, your microbiome composition all evolved to thrive on plants.

Animal products create an inflammatory burden. They require more metabolic energy to digest. They don't activate the metabolic cascades that plant-based foods activate.

For pure energy optimization, plant-based is biochemically superior.

WHY RAW WHEN POSSIBLE?

Raw foods preserve the biological systems that activate your metabolism.

Enzymes. Intact polyphenols. Metabolic recognition signals. Cellular structures. All present and active in raw foods. Many are compromised or destroyed in cooked foods.

Raw foods make your mitochondria work optimally.

But this matters when foods cannot be eaten raw (legumes, grains), gentle cooking preserves enough biological viability to provide excellent energy. The framework is not "raw or useless." It's "raw or whole and gently cooked."

WHY NO PROCESSED ADDITIVES?

Your cells don't recognize processed chemicals.

When you consume artificial colors, flavors, and preservatives your cells register them as foreign. Your immune system activates. Your detoxification systems activate. Your mitochondria shift from energy production to cellular defense.

You expend energy on processing the unrecognizable instead of producing the energy you need.

Clean food = lower metabolic burden = more available energy.

The Simple Daily Framework

This doesn't require complexity. Here's how to eat:

Breakfast:

Option 1: Raw fruit (unlimited) + raw nuts/seeds

Option 2: Whole grain (oatmeal, quinoa) + fruit

Option 3: Smoothie with raw fruit, raw seeds, plant milk

Lunch:

Large raw vegetable salad + cooked whole legumes or grains + herbs/spices

Dinner:

Large, cooked vegetables + cooked whole legumes or grains + fresh herbs

Snacks:

Raw vegetables, raw fruit, raw nuts/seeds as hunger dictates

Beverages:

Water, herbal tea, or fresh fruit/vegetable juices

That's it. No counting. No restriction. No deprivation. Just living foods in various states of preparation.

THE BIOLOGICAL TRUTH: WHY THIS WORKS

When you follow this framework, your body experiences something revolutionary:

Days 1–3: Your cells begin receiving the metabolic signals they evolved to recognize. Detoxification systems activate as processed substances leave your body. You might feel tired as your body reallocates energy toward cellular repair.

Days 4–7: Enzymes rebuild. Polyphenol signaling activates. Your mitochondria begin optimizing. Energy stabilizes. Withdrawal subsides.

Week 2: Glucose dysregulation ends. Your pancreas begins relaxing as it no longer needs to manage constant glucose spikes. Blood pressure begins normalizing. You feel noticeably better.

Week 3: Mental clarity emerges. Brain energy optimization proceeds. Mood stabilizes. Sleep quality improves. Inflammation reduces.

Week 4: Energy optimization plateau. Digestion adapts. Weight normalizes. You've entered the new normal where health becomes your baseline.

This isn't willpower. This isn't a restriction. This is your body responding to what it's been waiting for.

THE DISTINCTION: HOW THIS DIFFERS FROM OTHER APPROACHES

"Balanced diet" approaches try to mix living and dead foods. They balance processed with whole, expecting moderation to work. It doesn't. Your energy systems can't optimize when receiving mixed signals.

"Macronutrient optimization" approaches focus on protein ratios, carbohydrate percentages, fat calculations. They miss the point. It's not about the macro composition; it's about the metabolic activation the food provides.

"Calorie restriction" approaches limit quantity. Your body adapts by reducing energy production. You get tired and quit.

This protocol focuses on the quality of the signal your mitochondria receive. Unlimited living foods means unlimited metabolic activation. Your body thrives because it's receiving exactly what it evolved to thrive on.

THE ABUNDANCE, NOT DEPRIVATION

This is critical: The protocol feels like abundance, not restriction.

You eat unlimited vegetables. Unlimited fruits. Unlimited nuts and seeds (within reason, they're calorically dense, and your body signals satiety naturally). Unlimited cooked legumes and grains.

You're not saying "no" to food. You're saying "yes" to better food.

Compare this to every other health protocol:

- Low-carb diets: Restrict an entire macronutrient category
- Calorie restriction: Limit quantities constantly
- Macro optimization: Calculate and track every meal

Abundance creates sustainability. Restriction creates rebellion.

What Follows: The Journey Ahead

This chapter has introduced the protocol at a philosophical and practical level.

But introduction is not implementation.

The chapters that follow will provide the complete roadmap:

Chapter 6 will establish the 10 core principles that structure the protocol.

Chapter 7 will guide you step-by-step into implementation.

Chapter 8 will take you through the thirty-day reset with specific timelines and expectations.

Chapter 9 will show you how to measure your progress through medical markers.

Chapter 10 will troubleshoot obstacles you might encounter.

But first, you need to make a choice.

THE CHOICE: YOUR POWER AND RESPONSIBILITY

You now understand that:

1. **Your health is an energy system.** All function depends on energy availability.
2. **Your food is your primary fuel.** Food quality determines energy quality.
3. **Living foods create life energy.** Dead foods create only calories.
4. **One protocol addresses all disease.** All disease is energy dysfunction from the same root cause.
5. **Your body can heal.** Energy restoration is biochemically predictable and achievable.

You understand the Viability Principle. You know why living foods work. You see the framework.

But understanding changes nothing. Only action changes everything.

The choice is yours.

You can continue as you are. Continue disconnecting from natural alignment. Continue feeding your mitochondria dead matter and wondering why you're tired. Continue managing disease through medications instead of restoring health through natural foods.

Or, you can choose differently.

You can choose to trust nature's design over industry's profit motive. You can choose to feed your body living foods and witness the energy surge. You can choose to reverse your disease instead of managing it. You can choose to become an agent of your own health transformation.

This choice is your power. And with this power comes responsibility.

Your choices create your health. Your health creates your quality of life. Your transformation influences those around you. Your transformation contributes to a cultural shift toward natural alignment.

This is not a burden. This is FREEDOM.

The Bridge Complete

You've moved from philosophy to understanding. You understand why this protocol works. You know what foods pass the viable seed test. You see the distinction between life energy and calories.

The bridge from understanding to action begins in the next chapter.

The question is simple: Will you cross it?

Energy Restoration Protocol

Practical Implementation of the Energy Restoration Framework

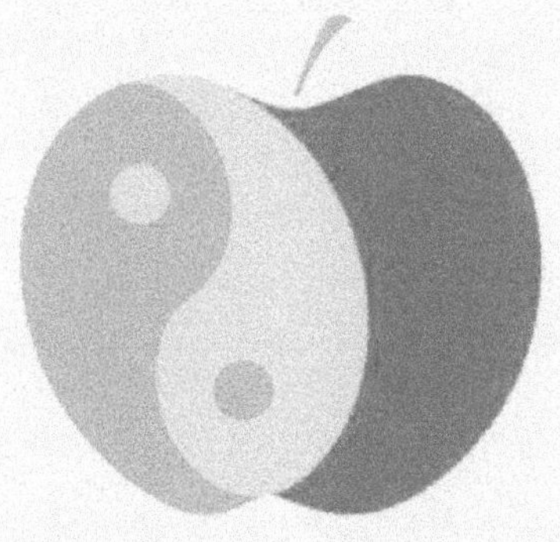

6

PROTOCOL FOUNDATIONS: PRINCIPLES OVER RULES

Introduction: From Restriction to Alignment

There's a fundamental difference between following rules and honoring principles. Rules are external, imposed, often arbitrary. They breed compliance out of fear or obligation. Principles, by contrast, are internal guides rooted in understanding. They create alignment because you comprehend the *why* beneath them.

This distinction matters enormously when it comes to restoring your energy system.

Most nutrition protocols fail not because the foods are wrong, but because they present themselves as a series of restrictive rules: "Don't eat this. Avoid that. Never have this again." The psychological weight of negation of deprivation eventually breaks almost everyone's commitment. We are not creatures wired for perpetual denial. We resist restrictions. We rebel against rules.

But we align with principles when we understand them.

This chapter isn't about teaching you ten rules to follow. It's about establishing the ten core principles that define energy restoration, so you understand not just *what* to eat, but *why* eating this way returns your body to biological alignment. Once you understand the principles, the food choices become obvious. They stop feeling like sacrifice and start feeling like wisdom.

The Energy Restoration Protocol rests on a simple foundation: your energy system is designed by millions of years of evolution to run on specific fuels. When you provide those fuels, your energy system optimizes. When you don't, it deteriorates. The ten principles that follow are simply expressions of this biological reality. They are not arbitrary rules. They are invitations to alignment.

Let's establish the principles, understand each one deeply, and then see how they translate into a daily life that energizes rather than exhausts you.

Principle 1: Whole Foods Only

WHAT IT IS

Whole foods are foods that have never been disassembled and reassembled. They exist in the form nature created them: an apple, a carrot, a grain of rice, a handful of almonds, a handful of beans. They may be cooked. They may be dried. But they remain structurally whole, their constituent parts have not been mechanically or chemically separated and recombined.

Processed foods, by contrast, have been taken apart (through milling, pressing, extraction) and often recombined with added substances to extend shelf life, enhance flavor, or speed absorption. A food that begins as whole wheat berries becomes "wheat flour" when milled, a crucial transformation that changes how your body processes it. A whole olive becomes "olive oil" when pressed, severed from the fiber, phytonutrients, and structural elements that made it whole.

WHY IT MATTERS FOR ENERGY RESTORATION

Your digestive system evolved to process whole foods. It recognizes the architecture of an intact carrot, its fiber, its cell structure, its enzyme inhibitors and responds appropriately, releasing the precise digestive secretions needed, pacing nutrient absorption, and signaling satiety. When you consume a whole apple, your body knows what to do with it.

But when you consume applesauce, apple juice, or dehydrated apple chips, something has changed. The fiber has been altered. The cell structure has been disrupted. The substance may still taste like an apple, but your digestive system encounters something different, something that requires a different metabolic response.

Whole foods are information rich. They carry embedded in their structure the metabolic instructions for how to be broken down and utilized. Processed foods are information depleted. They lack the cues that keep your energy system operating smoothly.

Most fundamentally, whole foods require metabolic work to digest and absorb. This work called the *thermic effect of food* is part of your body's energy maintenance. Processed foods slip through your digestive system with minimal metabolic friction, arriving in your bloodstream too quickly, triggering your energy system's emergency response mechanisms. The more whole your food, the more regulated and sustainable your energy.

WHAT IT PREVENTS

Consuming processed foods prevents your energy system from functioning as designed. It disrupts blood glucose regulation. It overwhelms your insulin response.

It deprives your cells of the micronutrients that fuel mitochondrial function. It leaves you feeling physically fed but energetically depleted, the classic symptom of processing-based nutrition.

WHAT IT ENABLES

Consuming only whole foods enables:

- Stable blood glucose patterns throughout the day
- Appropriate insulin response (not excessive surges)
- Micronutrient density (vitamins, minerals, phytonutrients that directly fuel mitochondria)
- Proper digestive function and nutrient absorption
- Genuine satiety (the signal that your body has received adequate nutrition)
- Sustained energy without crashes

HOW TO IMPLEMENT SIMPLY

Ask this question about every food: Could this exist in nature substantially as is? Some examples of putting this into practice include:

Apple Yes

Apple juice No (it requires extraction)

Almonds Yes

Almond butter with added oils and sweeteners No (it requires processing)

Chickpeas Yes

Chickpea-based snack crackers No

Brown rice Yes

Rice cereal No

This isn't complex. It's a recognition that you're consuming foods, not food-like substances. If it came from a plant or legume or grain and hasn't been mechanically or chemically disassembled, it is whole. Everything else exists in a sliding scale of processing, and the more processing, the less aligned with your energy system's design.

Principle 2: Raw Whenever Possible

WHAT IT IS

Raw foods are foods consumed in their uncooked state. This doesn't mean never cooking. It means recognizing that cooking changes food, and that when possible, especially for vegetables and fruits, consuming them raw maintains their structure and properties more completely.

WHY IT MATTERS FOR ENERGY RESTORATION

Heat changes food. It denatures some enzymes. It damages some heat-sensitive vitamins. It alters cell structure. Some of these changes are beneficial, cooking legumes and grains makes them digestible. But for fruits and vegetables, which humans have always eaten raw in nature, the uncooked state preserves the maximum biological information.

Consider an apple and how it is raw, contains enzymes, heat-sensitive vitamins, fiber structures, and cell walls that remain intact. When you bite into it, your digestive system processes these intact structures. When cooked, some of these elements are lost or altered. The apple is still nutritious, but it's less biologically complete.

More practically, raw foods retain maximum enzyme content. Enzymes are biological catalysts that facilitate the chemical reactions that produce cellular energy. By consuming foods with their enzymes intact, you're providing your mitochondria with pre-formed catalytic support. This is energetic efficiency.

WHAT IT PREVENTS

Consuming primarily cooked foods (when raw consumption is possible) prevents maximum enzyme availability. It also creates a subtle metabolic dependence; your digestive system exerts significant energy breaking down cooked foods that raw foods would break down partially through their own enzymatic action.

WHAT IT ENABLES

Consuming raw fruits and vegetables enables:

- Maximum enzyme availability (supporting cellular energy production)
- Preservation of heat-sensitive vitamins (particularly B vitamins and vitamin C)
- Intact phytonutrient structures (including polyphenols and other compounds that support mitochondrial function)
- Reduced digestive burden (the food's own enzymatic activity participates in digestion)
- Maximum bioavailability of minerals and micronutrients

HOW TO IMPLEMENT SIMPLY

Eat salads. Eat fruit. Eat vegetable snacks. Eat raw vegetable sides with meals. The principle isn't "never cook," it's "raw when possible." For every meal, ask "Can I include raw vegetables or fruit?" Usually, the answer is yes. For many foods, legumes, grains, and some root vegetables cooking is necessary for digestibility. But for the vegetables and fruits that form the foundation of your meals, raw is optimal.

Principle 3: Plant-Based Always

WHAT IT IS

Plant-based eating means deriving the vast majority of your calories, nutrients, and proteins from plants, such as vegetables, fruits, legumes, grains, nuts, and seeds. It means eliminating or dramatically minimizing animal products.

This doesn't require philosophical commitment to animal welfare (though that's valuable). It's a biological principle.

WHY IT MATTERS FOR ENERGY RESTORATION

Your energy system runs on glucose and ketones. Both are most efficiently and safely generated from plant foods. Plant foods provide:

- Carbohydrates that fuel immediate energy (glucose)
- Fiber that regulates energy release
- Phytonutrients that protect mitochondria
- Minerals that are cofactors in every energy production reaction
- Enzymes that catalyze energy metabolism

Animal products provide:

- Primarily saturated fat and cholesterol
- Concentrated protein (which requires significant metabolic processing)
- Compounds that increase inflammation and oxidative stress (countering energy production)
- No fiber (disrupting energy regulation)
- Heavy metabolic burden (requiring enormous digestive energy)

Most critically, animal products concentrate within themselves everything that the animal ate. If that animal ate processed grains, its tissues concentrate the inflammatory compounds from those grains, plus the animal's own inflammatory response compounds, plus cholesterol and saturated fat that increase vascular inflammation. Consuming animal products means consuming inflammation and metabolic dysfunction in concentrated form.[1]

Plant-based eating, conversely, means consuming the direct products of photosynthesis, the conversion of sunlight into biological energy. You're consuming energy that was captured directly from the sun and stored in plant tissue. This is energetically superior to consuming an animal that ate plants and converted that energy through an additional metabolic layer.

WHAT IT PREVENTS

Consuming animal products prevents:

- Optimal mitochondrial function (animal products contain compounds that impair mitochondrial efficiency)
- Efficient glucose metabolism (saturated fat impairs insulin sensitivity)[2]
- Vascular health (cholesterol and saturated fat damage endothelial function)[3]
- Rapid energy system restoration (animal products require the body to detoxify and clear them, diverting energy from repair)

WHAT IT ENABLES

Plant-based eating enables:

- Direct consumption of photosynthetic energy (foods that capture and store sunlight)
- Abundant phytonutrients (compounds that protect and optimize mitochondria)
- Optimal insulin sensitivity (plant foods contain fiber and compounds that regulate glucose metabolism)[4]
- Rapid inflammatory resolution (plant foods contain anti-inflammatory compounds)
- Efficient digestive function (plant foods contain fiber that your digestive system evolved to process)

HOW TO IMPLEMENT SIMPLY

Eliminate or minimize animal products. Most people transitioning find it easier to think in terms of what to add rather than what to remove, such as add more vegetables, more legumes, more whole grains, more nuts and seeds. As these foods increase to fill your plate and caloric needs, animal products naturally decrease.

Principle 4: No Refined Carbohydrates

WHAT IT IS

Refined carbohydrates are carbohydrate-containing foods where the fiber has been removed or altered, and the carbohydrate has been concentrated. White bread, white rice, pasta, pastries, crackers, and most cereals are refined carbohydrates. So are naturally sweet foods with fiber removed like fruit juice, dried fruit, and sweetened foods.

Whole carbohydrates are carbohydrate-containing foods where the fiber remains intact, such as brown rice, whole oats, legumes, vegetables, whole fruits.

WHY IT MATTERS FOR ENERGY RESTORATION

Refined carbohydrates enter your bloodstream rapidly, spiking blood glucose. Your pancreas responds with an insulin surge. Blood glucose crashes. Your adrenal glands release cortisol and adrenaline to raise blood glucose again. This rollercoaster repeated dozens of times daily is exhausting to your energy system.

Whole carbohydrates, containing fiber, enter your bloodstream gradually. Blood glucose rises steadily. Insulin responds appropriately. Blood glucose remains stable. Your energy system operates smoothly without emergency responses.

The mechanism is straightforward: fiber slows carbohydrate absorption, preventing glucose spikes. Glucose spikes trigger excessive insulin. Excessive insulin leads to glucose crashes, fatigue, mood disruption, and over time, insulin resistance the collapse of your energy system's ability to regulate glucose efficiently.

Refined carbohydrates were virtually unknown to humans throughout evolutionary history. They're a recent invention (refined flour, white sugar, and refined grain products are less than 200 years old). Your energy system has no metabolic machinery adapted to handling them efficiently. They overwhelm your glucose regulation system.

WHAT IT PREVENTS

Consuming refined carbohydrates prevents:

- Stable blood glucose (causing constant energy fluctuation)
- Appropriate insulin response (leading to eventual insulin resistance)
- Steady energy throughout the day (replaced by crashes and cravings)
- Optimal brain function (glucose instability impairs cognitive performance)
- Mitochondrial efficiency (swinging blood glucose impairs mitochondrial function)

WHAT IT ENABLES

Eliminating refined carbohydrates enables:

- Stable blood glucose throughout the day
- Appropriate insulin response (preserving insulin sensitivity)
- Consistent energy without crashes or cravings
- Clear cognitive function
- Optimal mitochondrial efficiency

HOW TO IMPLEMENT SIMPLY

Choose carbohydrates that still contain their fiber. Brown rice instead of white rice. Whole grain bread instead of white bread. Legumes instead of refined pasta. Whole fruit instead of juice. Oats instead of processed cereals. The principle is simple: If it's white, it's been refined. If it's brown, it's whole.

Principle 5: No Processed Additives

WHAT IT IS

Processed additives are substances added to foods for preservation, flavor enhancement, color, or texture.

This includes:

- Artificial sweeteners (aspartame, sucralose, and so on.)
- Preservatives (BHA, BHT, sodium benzoate)
- Flavor enhancers (MSG and its disguised forms)
- Emulsifiers (soy lecithin, carrageenan)
- Colorants (both artificial and "natural")

WHY IT MATTERS FOR ENERGY RESTORATION

Your mitochondria are exquisitely sensitive to toxins. Processed additives substances completely unknown to human metabolism require your liver to detoxify them. This detoxification diverts energy from other essential functions. Meanwhile, many additives directly impair mitochondrial function.

Specifically, artificial sweeteners disrupt gut microbiota, which regulate glucose metabolism and energy production. MSG and related compounds are excitotoxins that cause excessive neurological stimulation, including in your digestive nervous system, disrupting gut function. Preservatives and emulsifiers damage intestinal barrier integrity, triggering inflammation.

Your energy system can't optimize while your body is defending itself against chemical additives.

WHAT IT PREVENTS

Consuming processed additives prevents:

- Optimal gut microbiota function (essential for energy regulation)
- Intestinal barrier integrity (leading to chronic inflammation)
- Mitochondrial efficiency (your body expends energy detoxifying)
- Stable mood and energy (excitotoxins dysregulate neurotransmitter function)

WHAT IT ENABLES

Eliminating processed additives enables:

- Optimal gut microbiota function
- Intestinal barrier integrity
- Reduced detoxification burden
- Stable neurological and energetic function
- Rapid energy system restoration

HOW TO IMPLEMENT SIMPLY

Read ingredient lists. If an ingredient sounds like a chemical (rather than a food), it's an additive. Avoid it. Most whole foods have no ingredient list. An apple is an apple, lentils are lentils. When buying packaged foods (which you'll minimize as you align with Principles 1–4), choose products with ingredient lists you recognize and can pronounce.

Principle 6: No Extracted Oils

WHAT IT IS

Extracted oils are oils separated from their source foods through mechanical or chemical extraction: olive oil, coconut oil, vegetable oil, sesame oil, and all other bottled oils used in cooking.

WHY IT MATTERS FOR ENERGY RESTORATION

This principle surprises most people, so let's be precise about the reasoning.

Oils are calorie-dense but nutrient-sparse. An olive, whole, contains oil within a matrix of fiber, polyphenols, minerals, and other compounds. Your body processes the olive as an integrated whole. Olive oil, extracted from that matrix, is pure fat, all calories, no context.

More critically, extracted oils are oxidized fats, and oxidized fats impair mitochondrial function. The extraction process, storage, and especially heating of oils creates oxidative damage, the formation of compounds that directly damage mitochondrial membranes and impair energy production. Consuming extracted oils means consuming compounds that literally damage your energy-producing machinery.

Additionally, the molecular structure of extracted oils differs from the fats in whole foods. They're absorbed differently, processed differently, stored differently. They disrupt the carefully calibrated fat composition of your cell membranes and mitochondrial membranes, impairing their function.

This doesn't mean you won't consume fats you will, abundantly, from nuts, seeds, legumes, and whole foods. These fats are in their natural context, not oxidized and extracted.

WHAT IT PREVENTS

Consuming extracted oils prevents:

- Mitochondrial efficiency (oxidized fats damage mitochondrial function)
- Optimal cell membrane function (disrupted by non-native fat structures)
- Appropriate inflammatory response (extracted oils promote oxidative stress)

WHAT IT ENABLES

Eliminating extracted oils enables:

- Maximum mitochondrial efficiency
- Optimal cell membrane and mitochondrial membrane function
- Appropriate inflammatory response and resolution
- Rapid energy system restoration

HOW TO IMPLEMENT SIMPLY

Cook with water or broth. Roast vegetables without oil. Make salad dressings with whole food ingredients (nuts, seeds, plants) blended with water or vinegar, chutney, salsa. Get your fats from their whole food sources: nuts, seeds, avocados, olives, legumes. Your body will receive abundant fat just in the form it was designed to process.

Principle 7: Unlimited Vegetables

WHAT IT IS

Vegetables, especially nonstarchy vegetables like leafy greens, cruciferous vegetables (broccoli, cauliflower, kale), tomatoes, peppers, mushrooms, squash, and root vegetables, are so nutrient dense and energy supporting that the only guidance is more.

WHY IT MATTERS FOR ENERGY RESTORATION

Vegetables are literally the foundation of energy restoration. They contain:

- Minimal calories (so you can eat abundantly without excessive energy intake)
- Maximum micronutrients (minerals and vitamins that are cofactors in every energy production pathway)
- Maximum phytonutrients (compounds that protect mitochondria and support their function)

- Maximum fiber (regulating glucose absorption and supporting gut microbiota)
- Virtually no compounds that impair mitochondrial function

There is essentially no upper limit to vegetable consumption that would be counterproductive. A person eating unlimited vegetables, all else being equal, will restore their energy system more rapidly than someone consuming vegetables but also consuming other foods.

WHAT IT PREVENTS

Unlimited vegetable consumption prevents:

- Micronutrient deficiency
- Energy system malfunction
- Inflammatory processes that would impair restoration

WHAT IT ENABLES

Unlimited vegetable consumption enables:

- Maximum micronutrient density
- Maximum phytonutrient support
- Optimal gut function (through fiber)
- Rapid energy system restoration
- Satiety and satisfaction from abundant food

HOW TO IMPLEMENT SIMPLY

Aim for vegetables at every meal. Aim for a variety of different colors of vegetables containing different phytonutrients. Fill half your plate with vegetables. Snack on raw vegetables. Cook large batches of mixed vegetables for easy addition to meals throughout the week. The more vegetables, the better.

Principle 8: Abundant Fruits

WHAT IT IS

Fruits are carbohydrate-rich whole foods containing fiber, vitamins, minerals, and phytonutrients. Unlike fruit juice or dried fruit, whole fruits retain their fiber and maintain their structural integrity.

WHY IT MATTERS FOR ENERGY RESTORATION

Fruits provide carbohydrates in their most benign form: wrapped in fiber, accompanied by vitamins and minerals, in the form humans have consumed for millions of years. The fiber slows carbohydrate absorption, preventing glucose spikes. The carbohydrates themselves provide energy. The micronutrients support mitochondrial function.

Fruits are nature's energy delivery system: compressed sunlight, transformed into carbohydrate, fiber, vitamins, and minerals, all packaged to be consumed raw, digestible, and immediately available.

WHAT IT PREVENTS

Abundant fruit consumption prevents:

- Carbohydrate deficiency (which would impair immediate energy availability)
- Micronutrient deficiency
- Insufficient fiber

WHAT IT ENABLES

Abundant fruit consumption enables:

- Ready energy availability
- Satiety and satisfaction
- Micronutrient density
- Appropriate carbohydrate consumption for stable glucose and energy

HOW TO IMPLEMENT SIMPLY

Eat fruit. Eat a variety of fruits. Eat seasonal fruits. Eat fresh fruits as snacks and components of meals. Eat smoothies (blended whole fruit) when convenient. There's no practical upper limit to whole fruit consumption for most people.

Principle 9: Regular Legumes and Grains

WHAT IT IS

Legumes (beans, lentils, chickpeas, peas) and grains (rice, oats, quinoa, barley, millet) are whole plant foods containing carbohydrates, proteins, fiber, and micronutrients.

Unlike refined grains (white rice, white bread), whole grains and legumes retain their structure, fiber, and nutrient density.

WHY IT MATTERS FOR ENERGY RESTORATION

Legumes and grains have been staple foods for agricultural humans for thousands of years. Your digestive system evolved to efficiently process them. They provide:

- Sustained carbohydrate energy (through their fiber-wrapped carbohydrates)

- Plant-based protein
- Minerals and vitamins essential for energy production
- Fiber supporting gut health and glucose regulation

Legumes specifically contain compounds called enzyme inhibitors, which require cooking to break down. This is why legumes and grains are cooked (aligning with Principle 2: Raw Whenever Possible, but cooking is appropriate here).

WHAT IT PREVENTS

Regular legume and grain consumption prevents:

- Protein deficiency (on a plant-based diet, legumes are essential protein sources)
- Iron deficiency (legumes are excellent plant-based iron sources)
- Carbohydrate deficiency
- B-vitamin deficiency

WHAT IT ENABLES

Regular legume and grain consumption enables:

- Complete protein provision (legumes combined with grains and other plant foods provide all amino acids)
- Mineral and micronutrient density
- Sustained energy availability
- Full satiation and satisfaction

HOW TO IMPLEMENT SIMPLY

Include legumes or grains at most meals. Cook beans in batches and freeze in portions. Cook grains in batches and refrigerate. Include beans in salads, grain bowls, soups, and vegetable dishes. Rotate through different grains and legumes for variety. Aim for at least one portion of legumes or grains daily, often at multiple meals.

Principle 10: Daily Nuts and Seeds

WHAT IT IS

Nuts and seeds are whole foods containing plant-based proteins, fats, minerals (especially magnesium and zinc), vitamins, and phytonutrients. They include almonds, walnuts, sunflower seeds, pumpkin seeds, sesame seeds, flax seeds, chia seeds, and others.

WHY IT MATTERS FOR ENERGY RESTORATION

Nuts and seeds are extraordinarily nutrient-dense. A handful of almonds contains:

- Protein
- Fiber
- Magnesium (essential for mitochondrial function)
- Zinc (essential for immune function and metabolic rate)
- Vitamin E (antioxidant protecting mitochondria)
- Polyphenols (supporting mitochondrial function)

Consumed whole and unroasted, they provide all these nutrients in their natural form. They're calorie-dense but nutrient-rich, making them perfect for providing satiation and supporting energy while eating in abundance.

WHAT IT PREVENTS

Daily nut and seed consumption prevents:

- Magnesium deficiency (which impairs mitochondrial function and energy production)
- Protein deficiency
- Zinc deficiency

WHAT IT ENABLES

Daily nut and seed consumption enables:

- Optimal mineral intake
- Sustained satiation
- Nutrient density with minimal caloric burden
- Optimal metabolic function

HOW TO IMPLEMENT SIMPLY

Include a handful (about 1 ounce) of nuts or seeds daily. Add them to salads, to vegetable dishes, to smoothies. Eat them as snacks. Keep a variety on hand. Rotate through different nuts and seeds for different mineral and nutrient profiles.

The Principles in Daily Practice: A Simple Framework

These ten principles, when integrated into daily eating, create a pattern that looks like this:

Breakfast Example:

- Fresh berries (Principle 8)

- Oatmeal (Principle 9)
- Ground flax seeds (Principle 10)
- No oil, no additives (Principles 5 and 6)
- All whole food, plant-based (Principles 1 and 3)

Lunch Example:

- Large mixed green salad with raw vegetables (Principles 2 and 7)
- Chickpeas (Principle 9)
- Walnuts (Principle 10)
- Whole grain bread (Principles 4 and 9)
- All whole food, plant-based (Principles 1 and 3)
- No oil dressing (Principle 6)

Dinner Example:

- Roasted broccoli, carrots, and sweet potato (Principle 7)
- Black beans (Principle 9)
- Brown rice (Principles 4 and 9)
- Fresh herbs and spices (flavor from whole food sources, not additives; Principle 5)
- All whole food, plant-based (Principles 1 and 3)

Snacks:

- Fresh fruit (Principle 8)
- Raw vegetables (Principles 2 and 7)
- Handful of almonds (Principle 10)
- Herbal tea

Notice what's absent: extracted oils, refined carbohydrates, animal products, processed additives, or any foods that violate the principles. Notice what's abundant: vegetables, fruits, legumes, grains, nuts, and seeds are all whole foods supporting optimal energy production.

From Principles to Freedom

When you understand these principles, something shifts. You stop asking, "What can I eat?" and start understanding, "This aligns with my energy system's design, so I can eat it. This doesn't, so I won't." The principles become internal guides rather than external rules.

You also recognize immediately that these principles are non-negotiable for energy restoration. It's not that you *have to* avoid extracted oils, it's that if you want your mitochondria to function optimally, consuming oxidized fats will impede that. It's not that you *can't* eat refined carbohydrates, it's that if you eat them, you're choosing energy instability.

This reframing from "I have to" to "I'm choosing to support my energy system" is fundamental to long-term adherence. You're not restricting yourself. You're aligning yourself.

By the time you finish the thirty-day protocol based on these principles, these choices will feel normal. You'll have experienced directly how your energy, mood, cognition, and physical markers improve when you consistently honor these principles. Deviation from them will feel like choosing to undermine your own restoration.

The protocol works not because it's restrictive, but because it's aligned. The ten principles define the foods that support your biology, and avoiding everything else simply means you're no longer fighting your own design.

You're ready. The principles are clear. Your energy system's requirements are explicit. In the next chapter, we'll establish the practical pathway for implementing these principles, with specific guidance for your first week, your first month, and your first thirty days of restoration.

7

IMPLEMENTATION: STARTING YOUR ENERGY RESTORATION

Introduction: From Understanding to Action

You've now established the principles. You understand why your energy system requires whole foods, plant-based nutrition, and why processed additives, extracted oils, and refined carbohydrates impair mitochondrial function. You comprehend the *why* of energy restoration.

Understanding, however, is different from doing. Many people finish reading about optimal nutrition and then wonder: *Now what? How do I actually transition into this? What happens the first week? How do I handle cravings, social situations, my family's skepticism?*

This chapter bridges that gap. It's the practical architecture of implementing the specific pathway from your current eating patterns to full alignment with the ten principles of energy restoration.

We'll address:

- Medical preparation (knowing your baseline)
- Readiness assessment (deciding if now is the right time)
- Transition approach (all-in or gradual)
- Environmental preparation (pantry, planning, meal preparation)
- What to expect in Week 1 (withdrawal, adjustment, early wins)
- How to build sustainable habits in Weeks 2–4
- Support structures that ensure success

The goal of this chapter is to move you from understanding to confidence. By the end, you'll know precisely what to do, what to expect, and how to navigate the challenges that will arise.

Let's begin.

Part 1: Before You Begin—
Medical Preparation and Baseline

MEDICAL CONSULTATION FRAMEWORK

If you're currently managing any medical conditions or taking medications, consult with your health care provider before beginning this protocol. This isn't because the protocol is risky, quite the opposite. It is because restoring your energy system often improves your health markers dramatically, and your medications may need adjustment.

Specifically:

- **If you're taking diabetes medications (insulin, metformin, sulfonylureas)**: Your blood glucose may normalize rapidly on this protocol, potentially causing hypoglycemia if you continue previous medication doses. Your provider needs to monitor this carefully and adjust medications accordingly.
- **If you're taking blood pressure medication**: Blood pressure often normalizes within weeks on this protocol, requiring medication adjustment.
- **If you're taking cholesterol medication**: Your cholesterol markers may shift significantly as your body normalizes. Your provider should monitor this.
- **If you're taking thyroid medication**: Thyroid function often improves with restored energy system function, potentially requiring dose adjustment.

This isn't saying you should avoid the protocol to maintain medications. Rather, it's saying you should begin the protocol *with your provider's support*, so medications can be adjusted as your health improves. This is actually the ideal scenario your provider gets to witness and support your recovery rather than being surprised by improvements.

If your provider is unfamiliar with plant-based nutrition or seems resistant, consider finding a provider knowledgeable in this area. There are plant-based doctors, functional medicine providers, and others who understand energy restoration principles and can support your implementation effectively.

ESTABLISHING YOUR BASELINE

Before beginning, establish your baseline. This serves two purposes: (1) it gives you a starting point to measure progress, and (2) it provides medical markers that help guide your implementation.

Medical Baseline:

If you can, get the following labs done:

- Fasting glucose
- Postprandial glucose (glucose two hours after a meal)
- Hemoglobin A1c (average glucose over three months)
- Fasting insulin
- Lipid panel (total cholesterol, LDL, HDL, triglycerides)
- C-reactive protein (CRP inflammatory marker)
- Blood pressure
- Weight

If you can't access lab tests immediately, start anyway. You can establish baseline labs later. But if you can access them, do so. These markers will shift as your energy system restores, and tracking them provides concrete evidence of the protocol's effectiveness.

Subjective Baseline:

Beyond medical markers, track subjective experience:

- Energy level (rate 1–10 throughout the day)
- Sleep quality (hours and subjective quality, 1–10)
- Mood and emotional stability (1–10)
- Cognitive clarity (ability to focus, memory, mental speed)
- Physical symptoms (joint pain, digestive issues, headaches list any present)
- Cravings (what you crave most strongly)
- Hunger patterns (when you get hungry and intensity, 1–10)

Write these down. This becomes your comparison point. In two weeks, you'll refer back to this baseline and recognize the shifts in how you feel.

READINESS ASSESSMENT

Before committing to implementation, assess your readiness honestly.

Are you ready emotionally? Beginning this protocol requires commitment. You're changing your food patterns, which are deeply ingrained. Are you genuinely ready for this, or are you doing it because someone else suggested it? Genuine readiness intrinsic motivation is far more predictive of success than external pressure.

Do you have support? Ideally, you have at least one person (partner, friend, family member, or online community) who supports this protocol. If everyone in your household is skeptical or actively resistant, the protocol becomes harder (though not impossible). If you can't get full household support, at minimum identify one person you can check in with for encouragement.

Is now the right time? If you're in a period of extreme stress, traveling extensively, or going through major life changes, the protocol becomes harder. Not impossible, but harder. If possible, choose a relatively stable time to begin. However, don't use "not the perfect time" as an indefinite delay. The perfect time rarely arrives. If you're reasonably stable and ready, that's sufficient.

Are you clear on your motivation? Why are you doing this? Is it because you want more energy? Because you want to reverse a health condition? Because you want to feel better? Because you want to feel aligned with your values? Because you want to align with nature? Your specific motivation will sustain you through challenging moments. Get clear on it.

If you answer "yes" to genuine readiness, support, reasonable timing, and clear motivation, you're ready to implement.

Part 2: Transition Approach—All-In or Gradual?

People often ask, "Should I change everything immediately, or transition gradually?"

The honest answer is nuanced. Both approaches work. The question is which aligns with your personality and circumstances.

THE ALL-IN APPROACH

You immediately eliminate all nonaligned foods and shift entirely to the ten-principle protocol. Your pantry shifts from processed foods to whole foods. Your meals shift from animal products and extracted oils to plant-based whole foods. Complete transition over a period of days.

Advantages:

- Faster results (both metabolically and psychologically)
- Cleaner transition (no partial adherence creating confusion)
- Stronger commitment signal (you're all-in, which increases follow-through)
- Faster adaptation (your taste buds and cravings normalize more quickly)
- Faster energy system restoration (continuous alignment produces faster results)

Disadvantages:

- Withdrawal symptoms are more pronounced (many people experience headaches, fatigue, irritability in Days 1–3)

- Requires more upfront preparation (pantry clear-out, recipe knowledge, meal planning)
- Social challenges are more acute (if you're eating completely differently than others, it's more noticeable)
- May feel overwhelming (everything changes at once)

This approach is best for people who are highly motivated, have gone through previous dietary changes successfully, have supportive environments, or are struggling with significant health issues and need faster results.

THE GRADUAL APPROACH

You transition over two to four weeks, progressively eliminating nonaligned foods and adding aligned foods. Week 1 might focus on adding more vegetables and whole grains. Week 2 might eliminate processed foods. Week 3 might eliminate animal products. Week 4 might eliminate extracted oils. By Week 4, you're fully aligned.

Advantages:

- Gentler withdrawal (spread over time, withdrawal symptoms are less acute)
- Less overwhelming (you adjust to one set of changes before adding more)
- Easier socially (gradual change is less noticeable to others)
- More time to learn recipes and meal preparation
- Allows time to experience improvements as motivation

Disadvantages:

- Slower results (partial adherence produces slower metabolic shifts)
- Longer withdrawal period (spread out over weeks rather than concentrated)
- Risk of incomplete transition (some people get comfortable in the middle and don't fully transition)
- Takes longer for energy system restoration (continuous misalignment during transition slows restoration)

This approach is best for people who are less motivated initially, have previous experience with dietary setbacks, have unsupportive environments, or have mild health concerns and are less urgently motivated.

MY RECOMMENDATION

Honestly? If you can do all-in, do it. The concentrated discomfort of Days 1–3 is worth the rapid normalization that follows. Most people report that by Day 4–5, withdrawal symptoms begin subsiding. By Day 7, they're past the worst. By Day 14, they're experiencing clear improvements. The all-in approach front-loads the difficulty but delivers faster rewards.

However, if your personality or circumstances make gradual more realistic, then gradual is far better than perfect planning with no implementation. A gradual transition you fully complete is infinitely better than an all-in transition you abandon on Day 3.

Choose based on honest self-assessment: Which approach will you actually complete?

For purposes of this chapter, we'll address both in practical terms, but emphasize all-in preparation since it requires more upfront planning.

Part 3: Environmental Preparation

PANTRY REORGANIZATION

Your environment shapes your behavior. If your pantry is full of processed foods, extracted oils, and animal products, you'll eat them. If your pantry is full of whole foods aligned with the ten principles, you'll eat them.

Clear Out:

Go through your pantry and refrigerator. Identify foods that violate the ten principles:

- Processed foods (read labels for additives)
- Extracted oils
- Refined carbohydrates
- Animal products (if transitioning away from them)
- Foods you know trigger cravings

You don't necessarily need to throw them away (though you can). Some people donate them, give them to others, or consume them through the end of transition. But remove them from your immediate access. Don't keep temptations on your counter or in easily reached pantry spots.

Stock with:

Replace with whole foods aligned with the ten principles:

Vegetables (emphasis on variety):
- Leafy greens (spinach, kale, collards, lettuce)
- Cruciferous (broccoli, cauliflower, cabbage)
- Tomatoes, peppers, mushrooms

- Root vegetables (carrots, beets, parsnips, sweet potato)
- Squash, zucchini, green beans
- Store fresh and frozen

Fruits:

- Apples, berries, citrus, bananas
- Whatever's seasonal and local
- Store fresh and frozen

Legumes:

- Canned beans (for convenience)
- Dried beans (for economy)
- Lentils (quick cooking)
- Chickpeas, black beans, pinto beans, kidney beans
- Variety of options

Grains (Whole):

- Brown rice, wild rice
- Oats
- Quinoa
- Whole grain bread (minimal ingredients, no oil added)
- Barley, millet, farro
- Variety for rotation

Nuts and seeds:

- Almonds, walnuts, cashews, pistachio
- Sunflower seeds, pumpkin seeds, sesame seeds
- Flax seeds, chia seeds
- Variety for rotating

Seasonings and flavor:

- Sea salt
- Black pepper
- Garlic powder, onion powder
- Dried herbs (oregano, basil, thyme, rosemary)
- Fresh herbs (if accessible)
- Low-sodium tamari or coconut aminos (for soy-like flavor)
- Nutritional yeast (for cheesy flavor)
- Vinegars (balsamic, apple cider, rice)
- Spices (cumin, coriander, turmeric, paprika, cayenne)

Staples:

- Low-sodium vegetable broth
- Coconut
- Herbs and spices

Notice what's absent: extracted oils, animal products, processed foods, refined grains.

MEAL PLANNING AND BATCH PREPARATION

The second most important factor in successful implementation (after genuine commitment) is removing friction. The easier it is to eat aligned foods, the more consistently you'll eat them.

Meal Planning:

Plan your meals for the week ahead. This doesn't require elaborate planning. A simple approach is to choose two to three breakfasts, lunches, dinners, and snacks for the week and rotate through them,

Write them down. From this plan, create a shopping list. Shop once, mostly around the perimeter of the grocery store (where whole foods live) and the bulk sections (where legumes and grains are inexpensive).

Example Weekly Rotation:

Breakfast:

- Day 1, 4: Oatmeal with berries and walnuts
- Day 2, 5: Smoothie bowl (blended fruit with granola from ground nuts/ seeds)
- Day 3, 6: Whole grain toast with almond butter and banana
- Day 7: Fruit salad

Lunch:

- Day 1, 4: Chickpea salad (chickpeas, tomatoes, cucumber, herbs, lemon)
- Day 2, 5: Vegetable and black bean burrito bowl (rice, beans, vegetables, salsa)
- Day 3, 6: Lentil soup with whole grain bread
- Day 7: Leftover dinner

Dinner:

- Day 1, 4: Roasted vegetables with tofu-crumble (or skip tofu, just vegetables) and rice

- Day 2, 5: Pasta with marinara and white beans
- Day 3, 6: Stir-fried vegetables with tofu and quinoa
- Day 7: Something simple or restaurant

This rotation repeats, with variations as you learn and expand recipes.

BATCH COOKING FOR EFFICIENCY

The most powerful implementation tool is batch cooking, which is preparing food in quantity so you can easily assemble meals throughout the week.

Sunday Batch Cooking (2–3 hours):

1. Cook two to three types of grains in large batches. Portion into containers. Refrigerate or freeze.
2. Cook two to three types of legumes in large batches. Portion into containers. Refrigerate or freeze.
3. Roast or steam two to three types of vegetables in large batches. Portion into containers. Refrigerate.
4. Chop raw vegetables for salads. Store in containers.

Example:

- Cook brown rice, quinoa, and lentils
- Cook black beans and chickpeas
- Roast broccoli, sweet potato, and Brussels sprouts
- Chop lettuce, tomatoes, and cucumbers

Throughout the week, you assemble meals from these components:

- Monday lunch: chickpeas + roasted vegetables + brown rice + tahini dressing
- Tuesday lunch: black beans + chopped vegetables salad + whole grain bread
- Wednesday lunch: leftover lentils + roasted vegetables + quinoa

This reduces cooking from thirty to forty minutes daily to five to ten minutes assembling precooked components.

The First Week Investment:

Yes, batch cooking takes two to three hours on Sunday. But it saves you five to ten minutes every day for the next week. It removes the friction of "I don't have time to cook." It prevents the default to processed foods because you already have whole foods prepared.

This investment compounds. After a few weeks, you'll have refined your system, you'll be faster at batch cooking, and it becomes second nature. But in Week 1, plan for that two-to-three-hour investment as essential to success.

Part 4: Week 1—Transition and Early Adaptation

WHAT TO EXPECT: THE FIRST SEVENTY-TWO HOURS

When you shift to the ten-principle protocol (especially all-in), your body undergoes significant changes. Understanding what's normal helps you navigate it without panic or abandonment of the protocol.

Days 1–3: Withdrawal and Adjustment

If you've been consuming processed foods, extracted oils, and animal products regularly, your body has become habituated to them. Removing them triggers withdrawal symptoms, similar to other habit discontinuations.

Common experiences (Days 1–3):

- Headaches (often significant)
- Fatigue or low energy
- Irritability or mood changes
- Cravings (often intense)
- Sleep disruption (either difficulty sleeping or excessive sleepiness)
- Digestive changes (either constipation or diarrhea)
- Mild body aches or malaise

Your body is adjusting to:

- Absence of stimulants (caffeine from coffee, sugar spikes that create stimulation)
- Changes in your microbiota (bacteria in your gut are shifting from those that prefer processed foods to those that prefer whole foods)
- Inflammatory resolution (as processed foods are eliminated, inflammation begins to decrease, which can temporarily feel uncomfortable)
- Detoxification (your liver is processing the absence of its previous stimulation)

How to manage it:

- **Expect it and normalize it.** Knowing this is normal and temporary makes it far easier to navigate. Write it down: "Days 1–3, withdrawal symptoms are normal and will pass."

- **Stay hydrated.** Drink water consistently. Withdrawal headaches particularly respond to hydration.
- **Get adequate rest.** If you're fatigued, sleep. Your body is making significant metabolic changes.
- **Don't exercise strenuously.** Your energy is devoted to adaptation. This isn't the week to start an intense workout. Light activity is fine, but intensive exercise can amplify withdrawal symptoms.
- **Reach out for support.** If you're struggling, text a friend who's supporting you, or reach out to an online community. Knowing others experience the same thing helps.
- **Don't abandon the protocol.** The withdrawal passes. By Day 4–5, most symptoms begin subsiding. By Day 7, they're largely gone. If you deviate (eating processed foods or animal products) to relieve withdrawal symptoms, you restart the timeline. Stay the course through Day 3.

Days 4–7: Adjustment and Early Improvements

As your body adapts, withdrawal symptoms subside and you begin experiencing improvements.

Common experiences (Days 4–7):

- Headaches fade
- Energy stabilizes (often noticeably higher than before)
- Sleep improves
- Mental clarity increases
- Cravings decrease
- Digestive function normalizes
- Mood improves

By the end of Week 1, most people report feeling notably better. Fatigue is lifting. Clarity is increasing. They notice they're not crashing midafternoon anymore. Blood glucose is stabilizing.

Supporting this transition:

- **Celebrate improvements.** Notice and acknowledge what's shifting. Energy up? Say it. Sleep better? Notice it. These early wins sustain motivation.
- **Establish meal rhythm.** By the end of Week 1, you have a sense of how the protocol feels. You've prepared meals several times. You know what works for you.
- **Plan Week 2.** As Week 1 ends, plan Week 2 meals and shopping. This maintains momentum.

PRACTICAL WEEK 1 GUIDANCE

Breakfast Approach (choose one):

Option 1: Oatmeal with berries and walnuts (satisfying, warming)

Option 2: Smoothie of frozen fruit, plant-based milk, and seeds (quick, nutritious)

Option 3: Whole grain toast with almond butter and banana (simple, satisfying)

Breakfast provides stable morning energy and prevents midmorning crashes. Aim for oats or whole grain bread (Principle 9), fruit (Principle 8), and nuts/seeds (Principle 10).

Lunch Approach (choose one):

Option 1: Large salad with vegetables, beans, and whole grain (emphasis on Principles 7, 8, and 9)

Option 2: Grain bowl with roasted vegetables and legumes (Principles 7 and 9)

Option 3: Raw mix vegetables with chutney, salsa, hot sauce (Principles 1 and 9)

Lunch provides midday energy and prevents afternoon crashes. Emphasize vegetables and legumes for satiation.

Dinner Approach (choose one):

Option 1: Roasted vegetables with legumes and grain, herbs and spices (Principles 1, 7, and 9)

Option 2: Vegetable stir-fry with tofu and rice (Principles 1, 3, 7, and 9)

Option 3: Vegetable soup with beans and whole grain bread (Principles 1, 7, and 9)

Dinner provides evening satiation and supports stable sleep. Emphasize whole foods.

Snacks:

Fresh fruit (apple, berries, banana)

Raw vegetables (carrots, celery, bell pepper)

Handful of nuts or seeds

Herbal tea

Hydration:

Aim for water throughout the day. If you're a coffee or tea drinker, continue (but unsweetened). Herbal tea is excellent. Avoid sugary drinks, alcohol, and artificial sweeteners.

Part 5: Weeks 2–4—Building Sustainable Habits

WEEK 2: CONSOLIDATION AND CONFIDENCE

By Week 2, withdrawal is past. Early improvements are evident. The focus shifts from adaptation to consolidation turning this protocol into habitual practice.

What to focus on:

- Notice energy changes (you likely feel better, more stable)
- Experiment with recipes (try new vegetables, grains, legumes)
- Establish shopping rhythm (you now know what you need)
- Deepen support connections (if you have people supporting you, stay connected)

Practical focus: In Week 2, you're comfortable enough with the basics to begin experimenting. Try a new recipe. Try a new grain or legume. Vary your vegetables. This prevents monotony and keeps you engaged.

WEEK 3: DEEPENING AND REFINEMENT

By Week 3, the protocol feels normal. The food patterns are established. Your taste buds are normalizing to whole foods. Sweetness from fruit tastes normal rather than insufficiently sweet. You're not experiencing intense cravings.

What to focus on:

- Notice mental and physical improvements (cognitive clarity, emotional stability, sustained energy)
- Begin considering medical markers if you took a baseline (you might see early shifts)
- Address any obstacles that have emerged (we'll address this fully in Chapter 10)
- Deepen your why (reflect on why you're doing this and what's already shifting)

Practical focus: In Week 3, consolidate your understanding. You've lived this protocol for three weeks. You understand it experientially, not just intellectually. You know how you feel on whole foods. You know what happens when you deviate (even a small indulgence probably shows you the difference).

WEEK 4: INTEGRATION AND SUSTAINABILITY

By Week 4, you're thirty days in. The protocol is established. You're ready to consider this your new normal rather than a temporary experiment.

What to focus on:

- Notice how your energy is compared to baseline (write it down, compare to Week 1)
- Consider your medical markers if you established a baseline
- Identify what's working well (what meals do you love, what habits have stuck)
- Identify what needs refinement (if something isn't working, adjust it)

Practical focus: In Week 4, you're positioning for long-term success. You've proven you can do this for a month. You've likely experienced significant improvements. Now you're establishing this as your ongoing approach, not a temporary diet.

Part 6: Support Structures for Success

Implementation is easier with support. Consider establishing these structures.

COMMUNITY AND ACCOUNTABILITY

Ideally, you have people doing this with you (or supporting you doing it):

Option 1: Partner or Family Member

If someone in your household is also implementing the protocol, you support each other. You plan meals together. You cook together. You share experiences. This is powerful.

Option 2: Friends or Family Support

Even if people aren't implementing the protocol themselves, they can support you. Check in with them weekly. Share progress. Ask for encouragement. Real human support is invaluable.

Option 3: Online Community

There are online communities focused on plant-based nutrition and energy restoration. These communities provide support, recipes, troubleshooting, and encouragement. Consider finding and joining one.

Option 4: Professional Support

If you're struggling, consider working with a plant-based nutritionist or health coach who can provide personalized guidance.

CELEBRATION AND RECOGNITION

Small celebration of wins maintains motivation:

- Hit Day 7 without abandoning the protocol? Celebrate.

- Notice an energy increase? Acknowledge it.
- Sleep well for three nights? Recognize it.
- Month complete? Celebrate meaningfully.

These celebrations don't require expense or indulgence. They're recognition that you're changing your life, and that's worth noticing.

PRACTICAL TROUBLESHOOTING SUPPORT

Before problems fully develop, establish where you'll get help:

- If you have a health care provider supporting you, know when to contact them.
- If you have a nutritionist, schedule a check-in at Week 2.
- If you're in an online community, know how to ask questions there.
- If you have a friend supporting you, establish a check-in rhythm.

This prevents you from struggling in isolation.

Part 7: Decision Point—Are You Ready?

Before moving to Chapter 8 (the Thirty-Day Reset), pause and assess:

Do you understand the ten principles? (from Chapter 6)

Do you have a clear baseline (both medical and subjective)?

Have you chosen a transition approach (all-in or gradual)?

Have you prepared your environment (pantry reorganized, meal planned, batch cooking established)?

Do you understand what Week 1 will feel like (withdrawal, then improvement)?

Do you have support (at least one person or community)?

Are you genuinely committed to this for at least thirty days?

If you answer yes to all these, you're ready to move into the Thirty-Day Reset (Chapter 8), where we provide the specific structure, daily guidance, and medical marker tracking that will take you from implementation to transformation.

If you answer no to any of these, address it before moving forward. The protocol works, but it requires foundation. Take the time to build it now.

8

THE THIRTY-DAY RESET: YOUR ENERGY SYSTEM RESTORATION

Introduction: The Reset That Changes Everything

The next thirty days will transform you.

This isn't hyperbole. The thirty-day protocol is specifically designed to accomplish a complete energy system reset to take you from the dysregulation you've likely lived with for years (or decades) and restore you to a biological baseline in a concentrated period.

Why thirty days? Because this is the minimum time required for comprehensive restoration:

- Week 1 (Days 1–10): Your body removes the obstacles to energy production (detoxification, withdrawal resolution, energy stabilization).
- Week 2 (Days 11–20): Your body adapts metabolic machinery to new fuel sources (glucose normalization, insulin stabilization, initial marker improvement).
- Weeks 3–4 (Days 21–30): Your body consolidates the changes and establishes new baseline (complete physiological adaptation, vision for long-term sustainability).

By Day 30, you won't be a different person. But you'll be recognizably yourself clearer, more energetic, more stable returning to the baseline health your biology was designed to express.

This chapter provides the thirty-day structure, specific weekly expectations, daily guidance for what to do and what to expect, measurement frameworks so you can track your progress, and troubleshooting guidance for common obstacles.

By the end of this chapter, you'll understand exactly what your body will experience over the next month. You'll have concrete daily structure. And you'll have a measurement framework to recognize and celebrate the profound shifts happening within you.

Let's begin the reset.

The Thirty-Day Structure: Overview

The thirty-day protocol divides into three ten-day phases:

Phase 1 (Days 1–10): Detoxification and Stabilization

Focus: Remove obstacles, stabilize energy system, manage withdrawal

Marker: Withdrawal resolution, energy stabilization begins

Experience: Initial discomfort, then increasing clarity and energy

Phase 2 (Days 11–20): Adapatation and Optimization

Focus: Metabolic adaptation, marker normalization, deepening improvements

Marker: Blood glucose normalization, insulin begins responding appropriately

Experience: Marked improvements in energy, mood, sleep, physical symptoms

Phase 3 (Days 21–30): Consolidation and Vision

Focus: Habit consolidation, marker optimization, long-term sustainability planning

Marker: Complete physiological adaptation, baseline established

Experience: New normal feels normal, vision for permanent change clarity

Phase 1: Days 1–10—Detoxification and Energy System Stabilization

WHAT'S HAPPENING PHYSIOLOGICALLY (DAYS 1–10)

Your body is undergoing significant metabolic changes. Understanding the physiology helps you navigate the symptoms with confidence rather than fear.

Days 1–3: Removal of Stimulation, Withdrawal Begins

When you eliminate processed foods, extracted oils, and animal products (including dairy), you eliminate several stimulating compounds:

- Concentrated sugars (which create glucose spikes and energy surges)

- Salt in processed foods (which stimulates appetite and creates sensation)
- Omega-6 polyunsaturated fats (which create inflammatory stimulation)
- Certain compounds that trigger mild opioid-like responses in your brain (some processed foods contain compounds that create subtle addictive responses)

Without this stimulation, your baseline energy may initially feel lower. Additionally, your gut microbiota the bacteria in your digestive system begin shifting. The bacteria that thrived on processed foods (particularly those preferring high sugar and fat) begin dying off. The bacteria that thrive on whole plant foods (particularly those preferring fiber) begin proliferating. This shift in microbiota composition changes what compounds your gut produces and sends to your brain and body, creating the withdrawal-like symptoms described in Chapter 7.

Typical experience:

- Headaches (particularly Days 1–2, often severe)
- Fatigue or energy crashes (especially afternoons)
- Irritability or mood changes
- Sleep disruption
- Cravings (intense, particularly for sweet and salty foods)
- Possible mild body aches or malaise

Days 4–7: Withdrawal Resolution, Stabilization Begins

By Day 4, your body has largely processed the absence of stimulation. Withdrawal symptoms peak around Day 2–3 and then begin subsiding. Meanwhile, your body is beginning to stabilize on whole plant food fuel.

Specifically, your blood glucose is no longer spiking and crashing. Instead, it's rising gradually from meals, plateauing steadily, and declining gradually between meals. This stable glucose creates stable energy. No more energy surges followed by crashes. Instead, you have steady, sustainable energy.

Additionally, your insulin is beginning to respond appropriately to meals. Processed foods trigger massive insulin surges because refined carbohydrates hit your bloodstream rapidly. Whole plant foods trigger appropriate insulin responses because fiber-wrapped carbohydrates enter gradually. As your pancreas experiences this appropriate stimulus consistently, it begins to recalibrate.

Typical experience:

- Headaches resolving
- Energy stabilizing (no longer crashing midafternoon)

- Sleep improving
- Mental clarity beginning
- Cravings decreasing
- Mood stabilizing
- Early recognition that something is shifting

Days 8–10: Stabilization Deepens, Improvements Accelerate

By Day 8, you're largely through withdrawal. Your body has adjusted to new fuel sources. Your microbiota has largely shifted. Your blood glucose is operating smoothly. Your energy is stable.

In these final three days of Phase 1, you're experiencing the early benefits of a stabilized energy system with consistent energy throughout the day, improved sleep, improved mood, reduced cravings, and clearer thinking.

Typical experience:

- Stable energy throughout the day
- Improved sleep quality and duration
- Improved mood and emotional stability
- Reduced or resolved cravings
- Clearer thinking and focus
- Initial physical symptom improvement
- Growing confidence and motivation

Daily Guidance for Phase 1 (Days 1–10)

DAYS 1–3: EXPECT DISCOMFORT, EXPECT IT TO PASS

Your job in these three days is simple: consume the protocol foods, manage symptoms, and don't deviate.

What to do:

1. Eat according to the ten principles (Chapter 6). Every meal should have whole foods, be plant-based, and align with the protocol.
2. Hydrate extensively. Headaches especially respond to water. Aim for eight to ten glasses daily (or more).
3. Sleep as much as your body wants. If you're fatigued, rest. Your body is doing metabolic work.
4. Light activity only. Walk if you want to, but avoid strenuous exercise. Your energy is directed toward internal adaptation.

5. Reach out to your support person or community. Don't suffer in isolation.

6. Remember, this passes. By Day 4, things begin improving. By Day 7, you're mostly through it.

What not to do:

- Don't deviate, even slightly. Even one meal of processed foods restarts the withdrawal timeline.
- Don't overexercise. Your body needs energy for internal processes, not external exertion.
- Don't isolate yourself. Connection sustains you through this.
- Don't interpret symptoms as failure. Withdrawal symptoms are a sign your body is adjusting; this is success, not failure.

DAYS 4–7: RIDE THE IMPROVING WAVE

By Day 4, things are noticeably better. Your job now is to continue the protocol and notice the improvements.

What to do:

1. Continue the protocol perfectly. You're past the worst. Deviation now would only extend withdrawal.
2. Notice improvements. Energy steadier? Notice it. Sleep better? Acknowledge it. These observations fuel motivation.
3. Establish meal rhythm. You've now prepared and eaten protocol meals for several days. What patterns are working? What meals do you love?
4. Light activity beginning to feel good. If you want to take a longer walk or do gentle movement, it's appropriate now.
5. Share improvements with your support person. Celebrate that you're through the worst.

DAYS 8–10: CONSOLIDATE AND PLAN FORWARD

You've made it through Phase 1. Your body has stabilized on whole plant food fuel. You're experiencing marked improvements. The final three days of Phase 1 are about consolidation and planning.

What to do:

1. Continue the protocol (obviously).
2. Celebrate Phase 1 completion. You've done something significant.
3. Notice the improvements clearly and compared to Day 1. Write them down. This becomes your motivation for Phases 2 and 3.

4. Begin thinking about Phase 2. What would you like to focus on? (Often this is deepening meal enjoyment or beginning to measure medical markers.)

5. Plan your Phase 2 meals and shopping. Maintain momentum by looking forward.

WHAT TO MEASURE IN PHASE 1

Subjective measures (daily)

Rate these 1–10 each evening:

- Energy level (accounting for morning, afternoon, evening)
- Sleep quality (hours + subjective quality)
- Mood/emotional stability
- Mental clarity/focus
- Physical symptoms (any discomfort, pain, or specific symptoms improving or worsening)
- Cravings intensity

Write these down. Day 1 baseline is your comparison point.

Medical measures (if possible)

If you can measure at home:

- Blood glucose (if you have a glucometer)
- Blood pressure (if you have a monitor)
- Weight (though don't obsess over this; muscle weighs more than fat, so weight alone isn't complete information)

Most people won't have home measurement capacity. That's fine. If you took a baseline at a lab, you'll remeasure at Day 30.

Phase 2: Days 11–20—Adaptation and Optimization

WHAT'S HAPPENING PHYSIOLOGICALLY (DAYS 11–20)

Phase 2 is where the real transformation happens. Your body has stabilized. Now it's optimizing. Medical markers begin shifting dramatically.

Days 11–15: Glucose Normalization, Insulin Recalibration

Your body has now been consuming whole plant foods for ten or more days. Your blood glucose has been stable (not spiking) for ten or more days. Your pancreas has been receiving consistent, appropriate signals.

During this period, several things happen:

- Fasting blood glucose (glucose when you wake, before eating) begins normalizing.
- Postprandial glucose (glucose after meals) begins normalizing.
- Your pancreas's insulin response becomes more precise and efficient.
- Your cells' insulin sensitivity (their ability to respond to insulin) begins improving.

These shifts happen gradually over Days 11–15, but they're happening. Your energy continues improving because stable glucose creates stable energy. Your mood continues improving because glucose stability supports neurotransmitter function. Your mental clarity continues improving because your brain now has stable fuel.

Typical experience:

- Energy levels high and stable
- No afternoon crashes or fatigue
- Sleep excellent
- Mental clarity excellent
- Emotional stability excellent
- No cravings
- Physical improvements (reduced joint pain, improved digestion, and so on)
- Growing recognition that this is working

Days 16–20: Marker Optimization, Inflammation Resolution

By Days 16–20, glucose and insulin are normalizing. Additionally, your body is beginning to resolve inflammation.

Remember, processed foods, extracted oils, and animal products create oxidative stress and inflammation. Your body's constant work is defending against this inflammation. When you remove these foods, inflammation begins resolving. This resolution happens over weeks (not days), but it accelerates during Phase 2.

As inflammation resolves:

- Triglycerides (blood fat markers that increase with inflammation) begin dropping
- C-reactive protein (inflammatory marker) begins dropping
- Vascular inflammation begins resolving (meaning blood vessel function improves)
- Joint inflammation may resolve (pain decreases)
- Digestive inflammation may resolve (digestion improves, bloating decreases)
- Systemic inflammation resolves (overall sense of physical well-being improves)

Typical experience:

- All improvements from Days 11–15 continue and deepen
- Physical symptoms continuing to improve
- Weight beginning to normalize (as inflammation resolves and glucose stabilizes)
- Appearance improvements (clearer skin, brighter eyes, and so on)
- Clothes fitting differently
- Physical capacity increasing (you have more energy for activity)
- Mood high and stable
- Sense of genuine well-being

DAILY GUIDANCE FOR PHASE 2 (DAYS 11–20)

Days 11–15: Acknowledge and Celebrate Transformation

By Day 11, you're through the difficult phase. You're experiencing real improvements. Your job is to maintain protocol adherence and recognize what's happening.

What to do:

1. Continue the protocol perfectly. You're past adaptation now this is your new normal.
2. Notice improvements extensively. Energy compared to Day 1? Vastly improved. Sleep? Much better. Mood? Significantly improved. Cravings? Gone or minimal. Write it down.
3. Begin incorporating more movement if desired. Light exercise now feels good (walks, gentle yoga, swimming). Your body wants to move.
4. Experiment with recipes. By now you're comfortable with basic protocol meals. Try new recipes, new vegetables, new grains, new legume preparations.
5. Share your transformation with your support person(s). This reinforces commitment and provides accountability.
6. If you can, measure medical markers (blood glucose, blood pressure, weight). Early shifts are likely visible.

Days 16–20: Deepen and Extend

Days 16–20 are about deepening your connection to this way of eating and extending your physical improvements.

What to do:

1. Continue the protocol (obviously).
2. Reflect on changes so far. How different do you feel compared to Day 1? Write this down. It's powerful.

3. Incorporate movement you enjoy. If you like walking, walk. If you like dancing, dance. If you like cycling, cycle. Your increased energy supports physical activity.
4. Consider your long-term vision. Are you thinking about maintaining this permanently? Starting to envision a life where this is your normal? Spend time with this vision.
5. Deepen your understanding. Read about plant-based nutrition, energy restoration, or disease reversal. Learn more about why this is working.
6. Plan your Phase 3 focus. What do you want to accomplish in the final ten days? (Often this is establishing long-term meal patterns, planning a medical marker recheck, or beginning to consider disease-specific reversals.)

WHAT TO MEASURE IN PHASE 2

Subjective measures (every 2–3 days):

Continue rating:

- Energy level
- Sleep quality
- Mood/emotional stability
- Mental clarity
- Physical symptoms
- Cravings

Track changes. Most people will see significant improvement from Phase 1 to Phase 2.

Medical measures (Days 14–15 or 18–19):

If you can measure or get labs done:

- Blood glucose (fasting and/or postprandial)
- Blood pressure
- Weight
- If you can get a lab: lipids, glucose markers, CRP

Most people will see significant marker shifts by the middle of Phase 2. This is motivating.

Phase 3: Days 21–30—Consolidation and Vision

WHAT'S HAPPENING PHYSIOLOGICALLY (DAYS 21–30)

You're two-thirds of the way through the thirty-day reset. Your body has adapted. Your energy is restored. Your medical markers have shifted significantly. Phase 3 is about consolidation establishing this as your new baseline and envisioning permanent change.

Days 21–25: Physiological Consolidation, Habit Integration

By Day 21, all the major physiological adaptations have occurred. Your blood glucose is stable. Your insulin is responding appropriately. Your inflammation is significantly reduced. Your energy is high and stable. Your sleep is excellent. Your mood is stable.

During Days 21–25, these improvements consolidate. Your body settles into the new baseline. The protocol isn't new anymore, it's becoming normal. Meals that seemed special or different on Day 1 now feel ordinary. This is exactly what you want: the protocol becoming your default, your normal, rather than a temporary change.

Typical experience:

- All previous improvements stable and deepening
- The protocol feeling completely normal
- Cravings entirely gone or minimal
- Physical capacity high
- Appearance noticeably improved
- Medical markers significantly improved
- Sense of genuine health and well-being
- Growing confidence that this is permanent

Days 26–30: Vision Consolidation and Permanence Planning

The final five days are about recognizing the transformation that's occurred and planning for its permanence.

Over thirty days, you've experienced profound change. Your energy system has been restored. Your body's regulatory mechanisms have normalized. Your disease markers (if you had them) have shifted dramatically. You've lived this for a month and discovered it's sustainable and enjoyable.

Days 26–30 are about recognizing that this is who you are now, not a temporary experiment. Planning to make this permanent. Envision your life with stable energy, good health, and a clear mind as baseline rather than exception.

Typical experience:

- Recognition of profound transformation
- Confidence that this is permanent
- Excitement about long-term possibilities (health restoration, disease reversal, performance improvement)
- Integration of this as your new normal
- Beginning to think beyond Day 30 to the rest of your life

DAILY GUIDANCE FOR PHASE 3 (DAYS 21–30)

Days 21–25: Normalize and Deepen

By Day 21, you've proven you can do this for three weeks. Your job now is to deepen and begin integrating this as permanent.

What to do:

1. Continue the protocol (it's your baseline now, not a special effort).
2. Establish favorite meals and restaurants. By now you know which meals you love, which whole foods you prefer. Settle into these with contentment rather than constantly experimenting.
3. Physical activity at levels you enjoy. Your energy supports consistent activity. Incorporate movement that genuinely appeals to you.
4. Deepen community or accountability. If you're in a community, engage more. If you have a support person, continue check-ins. Share what you're experiencing.
5. Measure medical markers if you haven't recently. Most people will see substantial improvements. Let these fuel your vision of permanence.
6. Begin reading about or researching disease-specific applications. If you have a health condition, begin exploring how this protocol specifically addresses it (previewing Section 3).

Days 26–30: Consolidate and Plan Permanent Integration

The final week is about integration. You've done this for a month. You're not going back to your previous way of eating. You're planning forward into permanent change.

What to do:

1. Continue the protocol (your new normal).
2. Celebrate explicitly. You've accomplished something significant. A month of perfect protocol adherence is substantial. Recognize this.
3. Write a letter to yourself. Describe how you feel on Day 30 compared to Day 1. Describe your energy, your mental clarity, your physical improvements, your emotional stability. Describe your recognition that this is permanent. Describe your vision for your future on this protocol.
4. Measure medical markers if you haven't and compare to your Day 1 baseline. Most people see dramatic improvements. Write them down. These are your evidence.
5. Plan beyond thirty days. Will you continue the protocol? (The answer is almost always yes at this point.) Will you pursue disease-specific applications? Will you transition people in your life? Will you deepen community involvement? What's next?

6. Consider sharing your transformation. If you're comfortable, share your thirty-day journey with people who might benefit. Your story becomes evidence for others.

WHAT TO MEASURE IN PHASE 3

Subjective measures (weekly):

Rate overall:

- Energy level (steady, high)
- Sleep quality (excellent)
- Mood/emotional stability (stable)
- Mental clarity (excellent)
- Physical symptom improvements
- Overall sense of well-being

Compare to Day 1. The changes are profound.

Medical measures (around Day 30):

If possible, get the same labs you got at baseline:

- Fasting glucose
- Postprandial glucose (if possible)
- Hemoglobin A1c (this won't shift much in 30 days, but will shift over months)
- Fasting insulin
- Lipid panel
- CRP (inflammatory marker)
- Blood pressure
- Weight

Most people will see:

- Fasting glucose: decreased by 10–40 points (into normal range if elevated)
- Fasting insulin: decreased by 30–70 percent (dramatic reduction)
- Triglycerides: decreased by 30–50 percent
- Total cholesterol: may increase or decrease (total cholesterol is less important than particle type)
- CRP: decreased if elevated at baseline
- Blood pressure: decreased if elevated at baseline
- Weight: decreased by 5–15 pounds (depending on starting weight and point of focus)

These marker shifts are evidence of profound physiological change.

Timeline of Energy System Restoration: Physiological Detail

Below is a detailed timeline of what's happening in your energy system day by day:

Days 1–3: Withdrawal and detoxification begins

- Glucose spikes/crashes resolve as processed food is removed
- Insulin surges resolve as refined carbohydrates are removed
- Gut microbiota shift begins (bacteria die-off from lack of preferred sugar/fat)
- Withdrawal symptoms peak (headaches, fatigue, irritability)
- Energy system stabilization begins beneath symptoms

Days 4–7: Adaptation accelerates

- Withdrawal symptoms begin resolving
- Blood glucose stabilizes (no more spikes/crashes)
- Insulin response begins normalizing
- Gut microbiota shift accelerates (new bacteria proliferate)
- Energy stabilizes (no more afternoon crashes)
- Mental clarity beginning to emerge

Days 8–10: Stabilization complete, improvements evident

- Withdrawal largely resolved
- Blood glucose stable throughout day
- Insulin response normalized
- Gut microbiota shift substantially complete
- Energy stable and high
- Sleep quality excellent
- Mood stable
- Cravings largely resolved

Days 11–15: Glucose optimization, marker improvement begins

- Fasting blood glucose continues declining into normal range
- Postprandial glucose (after meals) normalizes
- Pancreatic insulin production becomes more efficient
- Cells' insulin sensitivity begins improving substantially
- Triglycerides begin declining
- Energy continues high and stable
- Physical symptom improvement (joint pain, bloating, and so on)

Days 16–20: Inflammation resolution accelerates

- All glucose markers continuing to normalize
- Insulin sensitivity substantially improved

- Triglycerides continue declining
- CRP (inflammatory marker) begins declining if elevated
- Vascular inflammation resolving
- Appearance improvements (clearer skin, brighter eyes)
- Weight beginning to normalize
- Physical capacity increasing
- Emotional well-being high

Days 21–25: Physiological consolidation

- All adaptations complete
- Energy system operating optimally on plant-based fuel
- Medical markers stabilized at improved levels
- Habit formation complete (protocol feels normal)
- Sleep excellent and consistent
- Mood stable and positive
- Physical health noticeably improved
- Cravings absent

Days 26–30: Vision consolidation and permanence planning

- All improvements stable and deepening
- Recognition of profound transformation
- Integration of protocol as permanent lifestyle
- Medical marker recheck showing sustained improvements
- Confidence in long-term sustainability
- Vision for future health clear

Measurement Framework: How To Track Your Progress

Measurement serves two purposes: (1) it provides objective evidence of change, and (2) it sustains motivation by making progress visible.

MEDICAL MARKERS TIMELINE AND EXPECTED CHANGES

Week 1–2:

- Fasting glucose: begins declining (may see ten-to-twenty-point drop)
- Postprandial glucose: begins normalizing (less dramatic spikes)
- Blood pressure: may begin declining if elevated

Week 2–3:

- Fasting insulin: begins declining substantially (30–50 percent drop common)

- Triglycerides: begin declining (10–20 percent drop)
- CRP: begins declining if elevated

Week 3–4:

- Most of above continue improving
- Weight: five-to-fifteen-pound loss common by Day 30
- Hemoglobin A1c: may not shift much in thirty days (reflects three-month average) but baseline for future improvement

SUBJECTIVE MEASUREMENT FRAMEWORK

Daily (evening) rating system:

Rate each 1–10:

1. Energy level (accounting for morning, midday, evening average them)
2. Sleep quality (hours + subjective quality)
3. Mental clarity/focus
4. Mood/emotional stability
5. Physical well-being (pain levels, bloating, general symptoms)
6. Cravings intensity (how much do you crave non-protocol foods)

Weekly summary (Sunday evening):

Review the week. How does this week compare to the previous week?

- Energy: Better? Much better? Stable high?
- Sleep: Better? Excellent?
- Clarity: Improving? Excellent?
- Mood: Stable? Elevated?
- Physical symptoms: Improving? Resolved?
- Cravings: Decreasing? Gone?

Thirty-Day Comparison:

On Day 30, compare to Day 1:

- Energy: How much higher? (most people report 50–100 percent improvement)
- Sleep: How much better? (most people report significantly better duration and quality)
- Clarity: How much clearer? (most people report dramatic improvement in focus)
- Mood: How much more stable? (most people report significantly improved emotional stability)

- Physical symptoms: How many resolved? (varies by starting condition)
- Cravings: How much decreased? (most people report cravings gone or minimal)

Troubleshooting Phase 1–3: Common Challenges and Solutions

Even with perfect protocol adherence, some people encounter challenges during the thirty-day reset. Here are the most common, with solutions:

CHALLENGE: PERSISTENT HUNGER

What's happening:

You feel hungry despite eating. This can happen if:

- You're not eating enough volume (whole foods are less calorie-dense than processed foods; you may need more volume).
- You're not including enough legumes/grains (protein and complex carbs from legumes provide satiation).
- You're including too much raw vegetables (without legumes/grains, volume alone doesn't satiate).

Solution:

- Increase legume/grain portion sizes at meals.
- Ensure every meal includes vegetables + legumes/grains + fruit or nuts.
- Add more nuts/seeds (calorie-dense, satisfying).
- Increase total meal volume if needed.

CHALLENGE: PERSISTENT FATIGUE (BEYOND PHASE 1)

What's happening:

You're through Phase 1 but still experiencing fatigue. This can happen if:

- You're not eating enough calories (whole plant foods require higher volume).
- You're exercising too strenuously during adaptation.
- You have an underlying condition (like iron deficiency) that's being revealed.

Solution:

- Ensure you're eating sufficient calories (aim for satiation at meals).
- Reduce exercise intensity; focus on consistency over intensity.

- Consider an iron supplement (plant-based iron is less bioavailable; some people benefit from supplementation during transition).
- See a health care provider if fatigue persists beyond Week 2.

CHALLENGE: BLOOD GLUCOSE NOT DECREASING QUICKLY

What's happening:

Your fasting glucose or other glucose markers aren't shifting as rapidly as you expected. This can happen if:

- You're still including some refined carbohydrates (hidden in products).
- You're still including animal products (which impair insulin sensitivity).
- You have underlying insulin resistance so severe that it takes longer to resolve.
- Your baseline was so dysregulated that the first improvements are subtle.

Solution:

- Review labels meticulously some products labeled "healthy" contain refined carbs or added oils.
- Ensure 100 percent protocol adherence (no animal products, no extracted oils, no additives).
- Be patient, deep insulin resistance takes longer to resolve, but it will.
- Consider a health care provider visit to ensure there's no underlying condition requiring additional support.

CHALLENGE: DIGESTIVE DISCOMFORT

What's happening:

You're experiencing bloating, gas, or digestive discomfort. This can happen if:

- Your digestive system is adapting to increased fiber (whole plant foods have much more fiber than processed foods).
- You're eating too much volume too quickly.
- You're not chewing food thoroughly (legumes and grains require thorough chewing).

Solution:

- Increase fiber gradually if just starting (though if all-in, this isn't possible; symptoms will pass).
- Ensure thorough chewing (aim for twenty to thirty chews per bite for legumes/grains).

- Include fermented foods (sauerkraut, kimchi, tempeh) to support beneficial bacteria.
- Drink adequate water.
- Symptoms typically resolve by Day 7–10 as your microbiota adjusts.

CHALLENGE: INADEQUATE WEIGHT LOSS

What's happening:

Weight is decreasing slower than expected, or not at all by Day 30. This can happen if:

- Calorie intake is still too high (whole foods have fewer calories than processed, but can still be overeaten).
- Exercise is building muscle faster than fat is decreasing (muscle weighs more than fat).
- You're retaining water due to high sodium intake (check salt levels).
- Your body is prioritizing other restorations over weight loss.

Solution:

- Track food intake for a week; ensure you're not overeating even on whole foods.
- Weight loss is not the primary goal health marker improvement is. If glucose, insulin, and inflammation are improving, weight will follow.
- If weight is truly stalled despite proper adherence, consider working with a health care provider or nutritionist.
- Remember, five to fifteen pounds in thirty days is a reasonable expectation; greater weight loss often indicates unsustainable practices.

The Thirty-Day Promise: What You'll Know by Day 30

When you complete the thirty-day reset, you'll know:

Your body is designed to run on whole plant foods. You'll have lived this for thirty days and experienced the difference. Your energy is higher. Your mind is clearer. Your body feels better. This isn't belief, this is direct experience.

Disease markers reverse rapidly when you align with your biology. If you track medical markers, you've seen them improve. If you tracked subjective markers, you've recognized profound change. Your body's healing capacity is more powerful than you expected.

Sustainable change doesn't require deprivation. You've eaten plenty of vegetables, fruits, legumes, grains, nuts, seeds. You haven't felt hungry or restricted. You've discovered this is abundance, not restriction.

Withdrawal passes. If you did all-in (or even gradual), you experienced withdrawal. It was uncomfortable. It passed. You survived it. You know you can do difficult things.

This is permanent. By Day 30, returning to your previous way of eating wouldn't make sense. You feel too good. Your energy is too high. Your body is too restored. This isn't a temporary protocol, this is your new normal.

Your vision for your future is clear. You're not wondering, "will this work?" You're not doubting "can I sustain this?" You're planning: "What's next? How do I deepen this? What health issues can I reverse?"

By Day 30, you've moved from understanding energy restoration intellectually to knowing it experientially. The abstract principles of Chapters 1–6 are now lived reality. The practical framework of Chapter 7 has become your normal. You've proven you can do this.

The next chapter teaches you to measure and interpret the medical markers that validate what you're already feeling. You'll understand precisely what's shifting inside your energy system, translating subjective improvement into objective medical evidence.

But first, complete your thirty days. Live the reset. Experience the transformation. By Day 30, everything will be clear.

9

MEDICAL MARKERS: MEASURING ENERGY RESTORATION

Introduction: Making the Invisible Visible

You've experienced the thirty-day reset. Your energy is transformed. Your sleep is better. Your mental clarity is sharper. Your mood is more stable. Your physical symptoms have improved. You know, directly and unmistakably, that something profound has shifted.

But knowing is one thing. *Measuring* is another.

This chapter is about translating what you've felt into what you can see medical markers that provide objective evidence of energy system restoration. Medical markers aren't arbitrary numbers on a lab report. They're measurements of your energy system's function. They show you, in quantifiable terms, exactly how much your body has healed.

Why does this matter? For several reasons:

Validation. When you see your blood glucose have normalized, or your triglycerides have dropped 40 percent, or your blood pressure has decreased 20 points, you have objective confirmation that your body is healing. This sustains long-term commitment.

Troubleshooting. If a marker isn't improving as expected, it provides information. Are you truly adherent to the protocol? Is there an underlying condition requiring additional support? This diagnostic power helps you optimize.

Communication. When you share your marker improvements with your health care provider, or with friends considering this protocol, you're not relying on subjective experience. You have data. Data is persuasive.

Long-term monitoring. Medical markers allow you to track not just the thirty-day reset but the months and years of sustained improvement that follow. You can monitor whether your improvements hold, continue, or plateau.

This chapter teaches you to understand your medical markers not as disease indicators, but as energy system measurements. It explains what each marker tells you about your energy system's function. It provides timelines for expected improvements. And it equips you to interpret your own markers and work effectively with health care providers.

Let's begin.

Understanding Markers as Energy System Measurements

Before diving into specific markers, we need to reframe how we think about medical markers.

Most medical education frames markers in terms of disease: High blood glucose means you're prediabetic or diabetic. High triglycerides mean you have metabolic syndrome. High blood pressure means you're hypertensive.

But this framing is backward. These markers aren't *names* of diseases. They're measurements of energy system dysfunction. They're the *evidence* that your energy system isn't producing, storing, and regulating energy correctly.

When we reframe markers as energy measurements, everything becomes clear:

Fasting glucose measures how well your energy system maintains stable energy overnight (your ability to produce glucose from stored reserves and keep it stable without eating).

Postprandial glucose measures how well your energy system responds to incoming carbohydrate food (your ability to take in glucose, transport it into cells, and store or utilize it).

Fasting insulin measures how hard your pancreas is working to maintain baseline glucose (if your pancreas is producing high insulin at rest, it's working overtime because your cells aren't responding to insulin efficiently).

Triglycerides measure how well your energy system is mobilizing stored fat for energy (high triglycerides mean your body is struggling to access and utilize stored energy).

LDL cholesterol measures vascular energy system function (oxidized LDL damages blood vessels, impairing their ability to deliver energy-rich blood to tissues).

HDL cholesterol measures your body's ability to clear excess cholesterol and transport lipids efficiently.

CRP (C-reactive protein) measures systemic inflammation (inflammation impairs mitochondrial function, reducing energy production).

Blood pressure measures vascular system energy efficiency (high blood pressure means your heart is working harder to deliver energy and oxygen to tissues).

Each marker, reframed, is a measurement of energy system function. When markers improve, your energy system is functioning better. When markers normalize, your energy system is functioning optimally.

This reframing is powerful because it removes the shame and disease-labeling that accompanies high markers. You're not "diseased." Your energy system is dysregulated. You're restoring its regulation.

Key Markers Explained: The Energy System Lens

GLUCOSE MARKERS: ENERGY AVAILABILITY AND REGULATION

Glucose is the primary fuel your cells use to produce energy. Glucose markers measure how well your body produces, regulates, and utilizes this fuel.

Fasting Glucose (FG)

What it measures: Blood glucose after eight-plus hours without food. This measures your baseline energy availability and your ability to maintain stable glucose overnight.

Why it matters for energy: When fasting glucose is high, your body is struggling to regulate baseline energy. Your liver is producing too much glucose (or your cells aren't responding to signals to stop). This dysregulation means you start your day already in an unstable energy state.

Optimal range: 70–100 mg/dL (some prefer 80–95)

Prediabetic range: 100–125 mg/dL

Diabetic range: 126+ mg/dL

Expected improvement timeline:

- Days 1–7: May begin declining if very elevated
- Week 2: Noticeable improvement common (ten-to-twenty-point drop)
- Week 3–4: Further improvement (often reaching optimal range)
- Months 2–3: Stabilization at optimal range

What it indicates about energy system:

- Optimal (70–100): Energy system regulating glucose efficiently

- High (100–125): Energy system struggling to maintain baseline; pancreas producing excess insulin
- Very high (126+): Severe energy system dysregulation; cells not responding to insulin appropriately

Postprandial Glucose (PPG)

What it measures: Blood glucose two hours after eating. This measures how well your energy system responds to incoming carbohydrates.

Why it matters for energy: When you eat, your blood glucose rises. Your pancreas releases insulin. Insulin carries glucose into cells. Glucose is utilized or stored. Blood glucose returns to baseline. This cycle happens dozens of times daily. If postprandial glucose spikes excessively, your energy system is overwhelmed by incoming carbohydrates. If it doesn't drop back to baseline, your cells aren't utilizing the glucose efficiently.

Optimal range: Below 140 mg/dL (ideally 100–140)

Prediabetic range: 140–199 mg/dL

Diabetic range: 200+ mg/dL

Expected improvement timeline:

- Days 1–3: Dramatic improvement (spikes may drop 50–100 points as refined carbs removed)
- Week 1: Substantial improvement; glucose curves become smooth rather than spiked
- Week 2–3: Further normalization
- Week 4: Stabilization in optimal range

What it indicates about energy system:

- Optimal (under 140): Cells responding appropriately to glucose; energy system processing meals well
- High (140–199): Cells not responding appropriately; glucose entering cells slowly
- Very high (200+): Severe cellular insulin resistance; glucose piling up in bloodstream

Hemoglobin A1c (HbA1c)

What it measures: Average blood glucose over the previous three months (glucose attaches to hemoglobin in red blood cells; higher average glucose = higher HbA1c).

Why it matters for energy: Fasting and postprandial glucose measure snapshots. HbA1c measures the three-month average of your sustained energy system function over weeks.

Optimal range: Below 5.7 percent

Prediabetic range: 5.7–6.4 percent

Diabetic range: 6.5 percent+

Expected improvement timeline:

- Month 1: Little change (HbA1c lags real-time improvement by weeks)
- Month 2–3: Noticeable improvement beginning (0.5–1 percent drop common)
- Month 3–6: Significant improvement (1–2 percent drop common)
- Month 6+: Stabilization at optimal level

What it indicates about energy system:

- Optimal (under 5.7 percent): Sustained stable glucose; energy system functioning optimally
- Prediabetic (5.7–6.4 percent): Sustained moderate dysregulation; averaging 100–140 mg/dL
- Diabetic (6.5 percent+): Sustained severe dysregulation; averaging above 140 mg/dL

Note on A1c: This marker improves more slowly than fasting glucose because it reflects past weeks' average. Don't be discouraged if A1c hasn't shifted much by Day 30. It will shift substantially by Month 3.

Fasting Insulin (FI)

What it measures: Insulin levels after eight-plus hours without food. This measures how hard your pancreas is working to maintain baseline glucose.

Why it matters for energy: Insulin is your pancreas's effort to manage glucose. If your cells are responding appropriately to insulin, your pancreas doesn't need to produce much insulin at baseline. If your cells are resistant to insulin (a condition called insulin resistance), your pancreas produces excessive insulin trying to force glucose into resistant cells. High fasting insulin indicates your energy system is working extremely hard just to maintain a baseline.

Optimal range: Below 5 mU/L (ideally 2–3)

Elevated: 5–10 mU/L

Significantly elevated: Above 10 mU/L

Expected improvement timeline:

- Week 1: Possible early improvement (20–30 percent drop)
- Week 2: Substantial improvement (30–60 percent drop common)
- Week 3–4: Further improvement (fasting insulin often normalizing)
- Month 2–3: Continued improvement; sustained normal range

What it indicates about energy system:

- Optimal (below 5): Cells responding efficiently to insulin; pancreas not working overtime
- Elevated (5–10): Insulin resistance developing or present; pancreas compensating with excess insulin
- Significantly elevated (10+): Severe insulin resistance; pancreas working maximally to manage glucose

Fasting insulin is often the most dramatic marker improvement. Many people see 50–70 percent drops within weeks. This reflects rapid improvement in cellular energy utilization.

LIPID MARKERS: ENERGY STORAGE AND MOBILIZATION

Lipids (fats) are stored energy. Lipid markers measure how well your body stores and mobilizes this energy.

Triglycerides (TG)

What it measures: Circulating fat in your bloodstream. This measures how well your energy system is mobilizing stored energy.

Why it matters for energy: When you eat carbohydrates, your body converts excess carbohydrates to triglycerides for storage. High triglycerides indicate your body is producing excess fat (because you're eating more carbohydrates, particularly refined carbohydrates, than you're utilizing). High triglycerides also indicate your body isn't efficiently mobilizing stored fat for energy between meals.

Optimal range: Below 150 mg/dL (ideally below 100)

Borderline high: 150–199 mg/dL

High: 200–499 mg/dL

Very high: 500+ mg/dL

Expected improvement timeline:

- Week 1–2: Modest improvement beginning (10–20 percent drop)
- Week 2–3: Substantial improvement (20–50 percent drop common)

- Week 3–4: Further improvement (often reaching optimal range)
- Month 2–3: Continued improvement; sustained optimal range

What it indicates about energy system:

- Optimal (below 100): Efficient energy mobilization; body not producing excess fat storage
- High (150–199): Energy dysregulation; excess carbohydrate intake relative to utilization
- Very high (500+): Severe dysregulation; often combined with very high glucose or severe insulin resistance

Triglycerides respond very rapidly to dietary change. Refined carbohydrate removal produces dramatic triglyceride improvement within weeks.

LDL Cholesterol (LDL-C)

What it measures: Low-density lipoprotein cholesterol. This measures cholesterol transport and vascular energy system function.

Why it matters for energy: LDL carries cholesterol from the liver to tissues. When LDL is oxidized (damaged by free radicals and inflammation), it damages blood vessel walls, impairing vascular function. Impaired vascular function means blood can't deliver oxygen and nutrients efficiently to tissues, reducing energy production.

Optimal range: Below 100 mg/dL (ideally below 70)

Borderline high: 100–129 mg/dL

High: 130–159 mg/dL

Very high: 160+ mg/dL

Expected improvement timeline:

- Week 1–4: Minimal change (LDL often doesn't change much in first month, or may increase temporarily)
- Month 2–3: May decline or increase slightly depending on individual factors
- Month 3–6: Stabilization; particle size often improves (small dense LDL becomes large buoyant LDL, which is less harmful)

Note on LDL: Total LDL number is less important than LDL particle size and LDL particle number. Small, dense LDL particles are damaging. Large, buoyant LDL particles are relatively benign. Plant-based diet increases LDL particle size, making LDL less atherogenic even if total number doesn't decrease.

What it indicates about energy system:

- Optimal (below 100): Efficient vascular energy delivery; minimal oxidation risk
- High (130–159): Vascular stress; increased inflammation and oxidation
- Very high (160+): Significant vascular stress; substantial energy delivery impairment

HDL Cholesterol (HDL-C)

What it measures: High-density lipoprotein cholesterol. This measures your body's ability to clear excess cholesterol and transport lipids efficiently.

Why it matters for energy: HDL is "cleanup" cholesterol. It removes excess cholesterol from tissues and blood vessels, transporting it to the liver for clearance. Higher HDL indicates more efficient lipid management and better vascular health.

Optimal range: Above 60 mg/dL (ideally 60–100+)

Borderline low: 40–59 mg/dL

Low: Below 40 mg/dL

Expected improvement timeline:

- Week 1–2: Possible early improvement (five-to-ten-point increase)
- Week 2–4: Continued improvement (ten-to-twenty-point increase common)
- Month 2–3: Stabilization at improved level

What it indicates about energy system:

- Optimal (above 60): Efficient lipid clearance; healthy vascular function
- Low (below 40): Impaired lipid clearance; vascular stress

Total Cholesterol (TC)

What it measures: Sum of all cholesterol (LDL + HDL + triglycerides/5).

Why it matters for energy: Total cholesterol is less important than individual components, but it provides an overall picture of lipid system function.

Optimal range: Below 200 mg/dL

Borderline high: 200–239 mg/dL

High: 240+ mg/dL

Expected improvement timeline:

- Varies by individual; depends on LDL and triglyceride changes

Important note: Total cholesterol can increase on a plant-based diet if HDL increases substantially (which is positive). Don't be concerned if total cholesterol increases while triglycerides decrease and HDL increases. That's an excellent lipid profile.

INFLAMMATORY MARKERS: ENERGY SYSTEM STRESS

Inflammation impairs mitochondrial function, reducing energy production. Inflammatory markers measure energy system stress.

C-Reactive Protein (CRP)

What it measures: Protein produced by the liver in response to inflammation throughout your body.

Why it matters for energy: Systemic inflammation indicates your energy system is under stress. Inflammatory compounds damage mitochondria. Removing them (through plant-based nutrition) allows mitochondria to recover and energy production to increase.

Optimal range: Below 1.0 mg/L (ideally below 0.5)

Borderline elevated: 1.0–3.0 mg/L

Elevated: 3.0+ mg/L

Expected improvement timeline:

- Week 1–2: Possible early improvement beginning
- Week 2–4: Noticeable improvement if elevated at baseline (30–50 percent drop common)
- Month 2–3: Continued improvement; stabilization at optimal range

What it indicates about energy system:

- Optimal (below 1.0): Minimal inflammation; energy production optimal
- Elevated (above 3.0): Significant inflammation; energy system under stress

OTHER MARKERS: ADDITIONAL ENERGY SYSTEM MEASUREMENTS

Blood Pressure (BP)

What it measures: Force of blood against blood vessel walls.

Why it matters for energy: Blood pressure is determined partly by vessel elasticity and partly by heart workload. High blood pressure indicates either stiff vessels (from inflammation and damage) or excessive heart workload (from energy system stress). When blood pressure normalizes, vessels are healthier and heart workload is reduced.

Optimal range: Below 120/80 mmHg

Elevated: 120–129/<80 mmHg

Stage 1 hypertension: 130–139/80–89 mmHg

Stage 2 hypertension: 140+ / 90+ mmHg

Expected improvement timeline:

- Week 1–2: Possible early improvement (five-to-ten-point drop)
- Week 2–4: Substantial improvement common (ten-to-twenty-point drop)
- Month 2–3: Continued improvement; often reaching optimal range

Note: If you're on blood pressure medication and it normalizes on this protocol, your provider may reduce or eliminate medication to prevent hypotension.

Weight and Body Composition

What it measures: Body weight and ratio of muscle to fat.

Why it matters for energy: Weight reduction reflects decreased inflammation and normalized glucose metabolism. More importantly, body composition (muscle versus fat) indicates metabolic efficiency. Increased muscle indicates higher metabolic rate and better energy production capacity.

Expected improvement timeline:

- Week 1: Possible initial weight loss (often water, as inflammation decreases)
- Week 2–4: Consistent weight loss (0.5–1.5 pounds per week common)
- Month 2–3: Continued weight loss until normalization
- Long-term: Weight stabilization at biologically appropriate level

Important: Don't obsess over weight. Weight is less important than how you feel, how your clothes fit, and your medical markers. Muscle weighs more than fat, so strength training combined with this protocol might show slower weight loss but better body composition.

Energy and Vitality (Subjective)

What it measures: Your subjective experience of energy throughout the day.

Why it matters for energy: This is the ultimate measurement. Everything else medical markers serve to support this: your lived experience of sustained, stable energy throughout your day.

Expected improvement timeline:

- Day 1–3: May dip as withdrawal occurs
- Day 4–7: Rapid improvement; energy stabilizing
- Week 2–4: Marked improvement; sustained high energy
- Long term: New baseline of sustained energy

Measurement: Rate daily 1–10. Most people move from baseline 4–5 (dysregulated energy with crashes) to 8–9 (sustained high energy).

Timeline of Marker Improvements: Comprehensive View

Here's a comprehensive timeline showing when you can expect to see marker changes:

Week 1

- Fasting glucose: May begin declining (if very elevated)
- Postprandial glucose: Dramatic improvement (spikes eliminated)
- Triglycerides: Possible early improvement beginning
- Blood pressure: Possible early improvement
- Energy: Improves by end of week

Week 2

- Fasting glucose: Noticeable improvement (ten-to-twenty-point drop)
- Postprandial glucose: Substantial improvement; normalized curves
- Fasting insulin: Dramatic improvement (20–60 percent drop common)
- Triglycerides: Substantial improvement (20–40 percent drop)
- Blood pressure: Noticeable improvement
- Energy: Marked improvement

Week 3

- All glucose markers: Approaching or reaching optimal range
- Fasting insulin: Often normalized
- Triglycerides: Often reaching optimal range
- CRP: Noticeable improvement if elevated
- Blood pressure: Often normalized
- Energy: Sustained high level

Week 4

- Most markers: Stable at improved levels
- HbA1c: Beginning to reflect improvements (but lags real-time)
- Weight: five-to-fifteen-pound loss common
- Energy: Sustained high, new baseline established

Month 2

- HbA1c: Noticeable improvement beginning (reflects Week 1–2 average)
- All other markers: Stable at improved levels or continuing to improve
- Weight: Continued normalization

Month 3

- HbA1c: Significant improvement (0.5–2 percent drop common)
- All markers: Stable at optimal levels
- Weight: Normalized for most people
- Long-term trajectory: Clear

Working with Health Care Providers

Your health care provider is your ally in this process, not an obstacle. Here's how to work effectively:

Before beginning (if possible)

Schedule a visit with your health provider. Tell your provider you're implementing a plant-based, whole-food protocol. Explain:

- You're eliminating processed foods, extracted oils, and animal products.
- You expect medical markers to improve.
- You want their support monitoring this and adjusting medications if needed.

Establish baseline markers by getting:

- Fasting glucose
- Postprandial glucose (if possible)
- Fasting insulin
- Lipid panel
- CRP
- Blood pressure
- Weight

During implementation

At Week 2–3 (optional): If you're on medications for glucose, blood pressure, or cholesterol, consider a check-in to see if markers are improving and medications need adjustment.

On Day 30: Recheck medical markers. Compare to baseline. Share improvements with your provider.

Communication

Be clear about adherence. When sharing results, make clear you're 100 percent adherent to the protocol. This helps your provider understand that improvements are from protocol adherence, not partial compliance.

Advocate for plant-based knowledge. If your provider is unfamiliar with plant-based nutrition, educate respectfully. Share research. Consider referring them to plant-based medical organizations (for example, American College of Lifestyle Medicine, Plantrician Project).

Medication adjustment is partnership. As markers improve and medications need reduction or elimination, work with your provider. Don't stop medications on your own, but do advocate for appropriate dose adjustment based on improved markers.

IF YOUR PROVIDER IS RESISTANT

If your provider is skeptical or resistant to plant-based nutrition:

- Ask what their concerns are specifically.
- Share peer-reviewed research supporting plant-based nutrition.
- Consider seeking a second opinion from a plant-based or functional medicine provider.
- Remember, you're the expert on your own body; your provider is the expert on medical science. Partnership is ideal.

Home Monitoring Tools: Tracking on Your Own

If you want to track markers at home:

Blood glucose monitoring:

- Home glucometer: Allows fasting and postprandial glucose measurement
- Cost: $30–50 for meter + strips ($0.50–2 per strip)
- Frequency: Test fasting daily for first thirty days; then weekly or as desired

Blood pressure monitoring:

- Home blood pressure monitor: Allows regular BP tracking
- Cost: $30–60
- Frequency: Daily for first thirty days; then weekly or as desired

Weight tracking:

- Home scale: Allows regular weight tracking
- Cost: $20–50
- Frequency: Weekly (daily weighing shows water fluctuation noise; weekly is clearer)

Lab work (professional):

- Baseline labs: $200–400 (varies by provider and what's included)
- Thirty-day recheck: $200–400
- Many providers offer this; functional medicine doctors often emphasize repeated marker tracking

Interpreting Your Own Markers

Once you have your markers, interpret them through the energy system lens:

Ask these questions:

1. "Has my glucose regulation improved?" (Compare fasting glucose and postprandial glucose)
2. "Is my pancreas working less hard?" (Compare fasting insulin the most dramatic improvement)
3. "Is my energy mobilization more efficient?" (Compare triglycerides)
4. "Is my vascular system healthier?" (Compare BP and lipid ratios)
5. "Has my inflammation decreased?" (Compare CRP if elevated)

Celebrate improvements. Don't compare yourself to others' markers. Compare to your own baseline. Your 20-point glucose drop is your success. Their 30-point drop is their success. Both are excellent.

Don't overfocus on single markers. Look at the overall pattern. If glucose improved dramatically but LDL increased slightly, that's excellent (you've improved glucose regulation; LDL changes don't negate that). If multiple markers improved, that's clear evidence your protocol is working.

Remember, marker improvements validate what you already know from lived experience. You feel better. Your energy is higher. Your markers confirm this. They're evidence, not verdict. The primary measure of success is how you feel.

The Marker-Experience Connection

Medical markers serve one fundamental purpose: they translate internal physiological change into external, measurable data.

You know, deeply, that something has shifted. Your energy is different. Your clarity is sharper. Your body feels better. You're not imagining that your mitochondria are producing more ATP. Your glucose is more stable. Your inflammation has decreased. Your cells are functioning better.

Medical markers simply make this visible. They show you the evidence. They allow you to know, not just feel, that your energy system has been restored.

By the end of thirty days, if you've tracked your markers, you'll have data proving that the energy system restoration isn't theoretical. It's real. It's measurable. It's yours.

This validation propels you forward. You're not relying on belief. You're relying on evidence. Your body has shown you, through improved markers and improved lived experience, that this works.

The next chapter addresses obstacles. Because even with improved markers and improved energy, real-world challenges will emerge. The chapter teaches you to anticipate and navigate these obstacles, so your long-term success isn't derailed by temporary challenges.

But first, measure your markers. Track your progress. Celebrate your improvements. You've earned them.

10

ADDRESSING OBSTACLES: STAYING ALIGNED WITH NATURE

Introduction: Real-World Implementation

You've completed your thirty-day reset. Your medical markers have improved. Your energy is restored. You feel better than you have in years.

Then real life happens.

Someone brings donuts to the office. Your family questions whether you're eating enough. You're traveling and the restaurants seem designed to avoid whole plant foods. You have a moment of intense craving. Work stress hits hard and you question whether you can maintain this while everything else is chaotic.

This is the reality of long-term protocol adherence: knowing the *why* and experiencing the *how* is profound, but navigating real-world obstacles is where commitment either strengthens or falters.

This chapter addresses the most common obstacles people encounter. For each, we'll explore three layers:

1. Understanding: What's actually happening? Why is this obstacle arising?
2. Immediate solution: What do you do right now, at this moment?
3. Deeper solution: How do you address the root cause so the obstacle doesn't keep recurring?

Additionally, for each obstacle, we'll address the perspective shift that transforms it from "problem" to "opportunity."

The obstacles are real. But they're also temporary. And they're all navigable. Let's address them.

Obstacle 1: Persistent Hunger

UNDERSTANDING WHAT'S HAPPENING

You're following the protocol perfectly, but you feel hungry. Not occasional hunger persistent, nagging hunger that doesn't go away despite eating.

This typically happens for one of three reasons:

Reason 1: Insufficient Calorie Intake Whole plant foods are less calorie-dense than processed foods. A processed meal might be 700 calories in two bites. A whole plant meal might be 400 calories in multiple servings. If you're eating the *volume* you're used to but switching to lower-calorie foods, you may be genuinely undereating.

Reason 2: Insufficient Protein or Complex Carbs Satiety comes from multiple sources: volume, protein, complex carbs, and fat. If your meals are heavy on vegetables but light on legumes/grains or nuts, you may not have enough protein or complex carbs to trigger satiety signals.

Reason 3: Habit-Based Hunger vs. Physiological Hunger You may have eaten in response to emotions or stress for so long that your hunger signals are disrupted. Your body isn't genuinely hungry, it's habituated to eating. This takes time to resolve.

Immediate Solution: Assess and Add

- **Increase legume/grain portions.** Add an extra serving of beans or rice to your lunch and dinner. Legumes provide protein; grains provide complex carbs. Both support satiation.
- **Add nuts or seeds.** A handful of almonds (about 160 calories) or seeds (about 150 calories) provides calorie density and satiation.
- **Increase total meal volume.** Don't be afraid to eat more vegetables. Fill your plate. Eat until genuinely satisfied, not just technically fed.

Deeper Solution: Understand Your Hunger

For insufficient calories, track food for three to five days. Write down everything you eat. Calculate calories. Most whole plant food diet recommendations are 1,800–2,500 calories depending on size and activity level. If you're eating 1,400 calories daily, you're undereating. Increase portion sizes until you reach 1,800+ calories.

For insufficient protein/carbs, ensure every meal contains:

- A source of legumes or grains (beans, lentils, rice, oats, quinoa)
- A source of vegetables
- A source of nuts/seeds or fruit

This combination provides protein, complex carbs, fiber, and healthy fat everything needed for satiation.

For habit-based hunger, distinguish physiological from habitual hunger. Physiological hunger is when your stomach genuinely needs fuel. Habitual hunger is when you're bored, stressed, or used to eating at a certain time. For habitual hunger, drink water or herbal tea. Often, the hunger passes. If it persists for more than fifteen minutes, it's physiological and you should eat.

Perspective Shift

Hunger isn't failure. It's information. Your body is telling you it needs more fuel or different fuel. Listen to it. Adjust. Hunger that leads to appropriate adjustment is your body working as designed. The goal isn't to never feel hunger, it's to understand and appropriately respond to it.

Obstacle 2: Persistent Fatigue (Beyond Phase 1)

UNDERSTANDING WHAT'S HAPPENING

You're through Week 1. Withdrawal has passed. But you're still experiencing fatigue. Not the deep tiredness of Days 1–3, but consistent low energy despite adequate sleep.

This typically happens for one of three reasons:

Reason 1: Insufficient Calorie or Nutrient Intake Your body requires adequate calories to produce energy. If you're undereating (see Obstacle 1), your mitochondria don't have adequate fuel. Additionally, specific nutrients (iron, B12, carbohydrates) are essential for energy production.

Reason 2: Excessive Exercise During Adaptation If you're exercising strenuously while your body is adapting to new fuel sources, your energy is divided. Your body is metabolically adjusting *and* expending energy on exercise. This creates a net energy deficit.

Reason 3: Underlying Condition Revealed Sometimes, the protocol reveals an underlying condition that needs additional support. Iron deficiency, vitamin B12 deficiency, or thyroid dysfunction can cause fatigue. As your body normalizes, these deficiencies become apparent because your body isn't masked by the fog of dysregulation.

Immediate Solution

- **Increase calorie and nutrient intake.** (See Obstacle 1 solutions.)

- **Reduce exercise intensity.** This isn't forever. After Week 2–3, exercise becomes beneficial. But during adaptation, gentle activity is ideal. Swap HIIT workouts for walks. Swap intense strength training for gentle yoga.
- **Get adequate sleep.** Your body is doing metabolic work. It needs rest. Aim for seven to nine hours. If you're fatigued, more sleep is appropriate.

Deeper Solution

For calorie/nutrient insufficiency, track calories and key nutrients for one week. Use an app like Cronometer (designed for plant-based diets). Ensure you're getting:

- Adequate calories (1,800–2,500+ depending on size)
- Adequate protein (50–100g depending on body size)
- Adequate iron (plant-based iron is less bioavailable; 18 mg daily for women, 8 mg for men)
- Adequate B12 (plant-based sources are limited; supplement 25–100 mcg daily or get lab-confirmed status)

For excessive exercise, exercise three to four times per week for thirty to forty-five minutes at moderate intensity (you can talk but not sing during exercise). Avoid intense exercise until Week 3–4 when your energy is more stable.

For underlying condition, see a health care provider. Get labs checking:

- Ferritin (iron stores)
- B12 and methylmalonic acid (B12 status)
- Thyroid panel (TSH, free T4, free T3)
- Complete blood count (CBC checks for anemia)

If any are deficient, supplementation or dietary adjustment can restore energy.

Perspective Shift

Fatigue that persists beyond Week 1–2 isn't normal or necessary. It's information that something needs adjustment. Respond to it. Increase food. Decrease exercise. See a provider. Your energy should be notably higher by Week 2. If it isn't, something needs addressing. Fatigue isn't the price of health, it's the signal that health restoration isn't complete yet.

Obstacle 3: Blood Glucose Not Decreasing Quickly

UNDERSTANDING WHAT'S HAPPENING

You're following the protocol. Your energy is better. But your fasting glucose or postprandial glucose hasn't decreased as much as you expected, or as much as others report.

This typically happens for one of three reasons:

Reason 1: Hidden Refined Carbohydrates or Processed Foods Some foods labeled "healthy" contain refined carbohydrates or additives. Whole wheat bread with added oils. "Natural" granola bars with refined sugars. Health food bars with extracted oils. These subtly undermine glucose stabilization.

Reason 2: Non-Protocol Foods Still Present You're 95 percent adherent but occasionally eating animal products, extracted oils, or processed foods. This 5 percent nonadherence, repeated regularly, prevents complete glucose normalization.

Reason 3: Underlying Insulin Resistance So Severe It Requires Longer to Resolve Some people have such profound insulin resistance (often from decades of dysregulation) that glucose normalization takes weeks or months rather than days. The protocol is working, but the baseline dysfunction was more severe.

Immediate Solution

- **Read every label meticulously.** Check for added oils and sugars, refined carbohydrates, and additives. If you can't recognize the ingredient, question whether it violates the ten principles.
- **Return to simple foods.** For one week, eat only foods with zero question marks, such as vegetables, fruits, legumes, whole grains, nuts, seeds. Nothing packaged. Nothing with ingredient lists. This resets your baseline.
- **Consider individual factors.** Some people with PCOS (polycystic ovary syndrome) or other hormonal conditions require lower carbohydrate loads. If glucose isn't improving despite protocol adherence, you may need personalized adjustment.

Deeper Solution

For hidden refined carbs, spend a week documenting everything. Check labels obsessively. You may discover "whole grain bread" is actually 40 percent refined flour. You may find "natural granola" has 15g of sugar per serving. Once you identify the culprits, eliminate them.

For non-protocol adherence, commit explicitly to 100 percent adherence for fourteen days. Not 95 percent. Not 90 percent. 100 percent. No animal products. No extracted oils. No processed foods. After fourteen days of perfect adherence, reassess glucose markers. The difference is usually obvious.

For severe underlying insulin resistance, know this isn't failure. It's a normal variation. Your glucose will normalize; it just takes longer. Continue perfect protocol adherence. Recheck markers at Week 6 instead of Week 4. Insulin resistance that took twenty years to develop may take six to twelve weeks to resolve. That's still extraordinarily fast compared to the lifetime dysfunction without intervention.

Perspective Shift

Slower glucose normalization isn't personal failure, it's information about your baseline dysfunction severity. Someone with moderate insulin resistance might see dramatic improvement in two weeks. Someone with severe insulin resistance might take six weeks. Both are succeeding. Both are healing. One is just starting from a deeper hole. Continue the protocol. Trust the process. The markers will normalize. It may just take a bit longer.

Obstacle 4: Digestive Discomfort

UNDERSTANDING WHAT'S HAPPENING

You're experiencing bloating, gas, constipation, or diarrhea. Your digestive system is unhappy.

This typically happens for one of three reasons:

Reason 1: Rapid Fiber Increase Whole plant foods contain far more fiber than processed foods. Your gut bacteria haven't adapted yet. They're fermenting the increase in fiber, creating gas. Your colon is working harder to move bulk through, creating bloating.

Reason 2: Inadequate Hydration Fiber requires water to move through your digestive system. If you're increasing fiber but not increasing water, you get constipation or sluggish digestion.

Reason 3: Insufficient Chewing or Rushing Meals Legumes and grains require thorough chewing to break them down adequately. If you're swallowing large pieces, your digestive system works harder, creating gas and discomfort.

Immediate Solution

- **Hydrate extensively.** Drink eight to ten glasses of water daily. Herbal tea counts. Water is essential for fiber movement.
- **Chew thoroughly.** Aim for twenty to thirty chews per bite, especially legumes and grains. You're not in a hurry. Chewing is the beginning of digestion.
- **Include fermented foods.** Sauerkraut, kimchi, miso, tempeh these support beneficial bacteria and ease transition. A few tablespoons daily helps.

Deeper Solution

For fiber adaptation, if you did all-in transition, your symptoms will peak around Day 2–3 and resolve by Day 7–10. If you do a gradual transition, increase fiber more slowly. If you're past Day 10 and still experiencing significant gas/bloating, see a health care provider to rule out conditions like FODMAP sensitivity or SIBO (small intestinal bacterial overgrowth).

For constipation, increase water intake to twelve or more glasses daily. If still constipated after three days, add ground flaxseed (1–2 tablespoons mixed in water or food daily) or psyllium husk (follow package directions). Both increase bulk and support bowel movement.

For diarrhea, this often resolves as your system adapts. If persistent beyond Day 10, reduce raw vegetables temporarily (eat more cooked vegetables). Increase soluble fiber (oatmeal, fruit) relative to insoluble fiber (leafy greens). Reintroduce raw vegetables gradually once diarrhea resolves.

Perspective Shift

Digestive discomfort during transition is normal and temporary. It's not a sign something is wrong; it's a sign your digestive system is adapting to real food after years of processed food. You're not breaking. Your gut bacteria are shifting. Your digestive organs are relearning. This is healing, even when uncomfortable. Push through. By Day 10, most digestive discomfort resolves, and you're left with superior digestive function.

Obstacle 5: Inadequate Weight Loss

UNDERSTANDING WHAT'S HAPPENING

You've been on the protocol for thirty days. You feel good. Your medical markers have improved. But the scale isn't moving as much as you expected.

This typically happens for one of three reasons:

Reason 1: Muscle Gain Offsetting Fat Loss If you're exercising (especially strength training) while losing fat, you're gaining muscle. Muscle weighs more than fat. Scale weight may stay the same or increase while body composition is improving.

Reason 2: Calorie Intake Still Slightly Elevated It's possible to overeat whole foods. A handful of nuts is 200 calories. Four handfuls is 800 calories. If you're eating abundantly but also exceeding caloric needs, weight loss slows.

Reason 3: Your Body Prioritizing Other Health Restorations Sometimes, your body prioritizes resolving inflammation, stabilizing hormones, or restoring metabolic function before significant weight loss occurs. This is actually a sign of deep healing. Your body is doing foundational restoration.

Immediate Solution

- **Measure body composition, not just weight.** How do your clothes fit? How do you look in the mirror? Have measurements at waist, hip, chest changed? These are more meaningful than scale weight.
- **Focus on how you feel.** More important than weight loss is how your energy, mood, and physical function have improved. You've succeeded regardless of scale movement.
- **Be patient.** Weight normalization is the ultimate outcome of sustained protocol adherence. It may take two to three months instead of thirty days. That's still remarkably fast.

Deeper Solution

Muscle gain offsetting fat loss is actually excellent. Muscle tissue is metabolically active. More muscle means higher metabolic rate and better energy production capacity. Celebrate this. Your body is becoming stronger and more efficient.

For slightly elevated calorie intake, track for one week. If you're exceeding your caloric needs by 200–300 calories daily, slightly reduce portion sizes. But don't drastically cut calories, you need adequate fuel for energy production. A modest calorie reduction (100–200 daily) is appropriate; severe restriction is counterproductive.

The body prioritizing other restoration is profound healing. Your body knows what it needs. If weight loss is slower but all other markers are improving, your body is healing foundationally. Weight loss will follow. Continue protocol adherence.

Perspective Shift

Weight is the least important marker of health restoration. Yes, normalization of weight is a goal. But it's not the primary goal. Primary goals are stable energy, clear mind, resolved symptoms, and normalized medical markers. Weight loss follows these. If you have abundant energy, normalized glucose, decreased inflammation, and excellent mood but scale weight is moving slowly, you're winning. The weight will come. Your body knows how.

Obstacle 6: Social Pressure and Isolation

UNDERSTANDING WHAT'S HAPPENING

Your family questions your diet. Your friends don't understand why you won't eat their food. People at social gatherings comment, question, or actively pressure you to deviate. You feel isolated, everyone else eating differently, you standing alone.

This is real, and it's one of the most underestimated obstacles to long-term adherence.

Root causes:

- People fear what they don't understand
- People's dietary choices feel personally challenged by your choice
- Food is deeply cultural and social
- Deviation from group norms creates tension

Immediate Solution

- **Find your people.** Connect with others following similar protocols online communities, local groups, or individuals. Knowing others are doing this sustains you.
- **Set boundaries with compassion.** "I appreciate the offer, and I'm not eating animal products right now. I brought my own food/can eat before we go/can suggest a restaurant that works for me." Firm boundaries without defensiveness.
- **Lead with your results, not your words.** Don't evangelize. Just live visibly. Your improved energy and health speak louder than arguments.

Deeper Solution

For family pressure, have a genuine conversation. Explain you're doing this for your health. Share specific improvements (better energy, better sleep, resolved symptoms). Invite them to your appointments if they're skeptical. Invite them to try meals you're making many people convert when they taste the food. But ultimately, your health is your decision. Respectfully but firmly hold your boundary.

For cultural food traditions, you can honor traditions while adapting them. Indian cuisine has abundant plant-based options. Mediterranean cuisine is naturally plant heavy. Mexican cuisine can be entirely plant-based. Asian cuisines are often plant-forward. Find the plant-based expressions of your cultural foods.

For social isolation, expect it to be temporary. After two to three months, people adjust. They stop questioning. They recognize your commitment and accept it. Some may even become curious. In the meantime, find your community whether online or in-person. You're not alone.

Perspective Shift

Social pressure is normal and temporary. People fear what's unfamiliar. Your deviation from normal eating challenges their choices. This is their process to work through, not your responsibility. You're not responsible for making others comfortable with your health choices. What you *are* responsible for is your own health. Maintain boundaries compassionately. Connect with your people. Lead with your results. The isolation passes. On the other side are community people who understand and support you.

Obstacle 7: Restaurant and Travel Challenges

UNDERSTANDING WHAT'S HAPPENING

You're traveling or eating out regularly. The restaurants seem designed to include animal products, extracted oils, and processed ingredients in everything. You feel trapped between protocol adherence and practical impossibility.

Root causes:

- Standard restaurant cuisine is built on animal products and oils
- Many cuisines have few visible plant-based options
- You don't control food preparation
- Travel makes meal planning harder

Immediate Solution

- **Call ahead.** Before going to a restaurant, call and ask, "Can you prepare a meal with vegetables, grains, and legumes, no animal products, no oils?" Many restaurants will accommodate if asked in advance.
- **Know your cuisines.** Some restaurants make protocol adherence easy:
  - Thai: Vegetable curries (request no fish sauce, oil on side)
  - Indian: Dal, chickpea curries, vegetable dishes
  - Mexican: Bean burritos (ask for no cheese, oil), rice bowls
  - Italian: Pasta with marinara and vegetables (oil on side)
  - Chinese: Vegetable dishes (request no oil, soy sauce on side)
- **Eat before or after if needed.** If no good options exist, eat a substantial meal before you go. Participate socially without eating, or eat after. It's not ideal, but it's protocol-adherent.

Deeper Solution

For frequent restaurant eating, identify two to three restaurants where you regularly eat. Build relationships with them. Tell them your dietary needs. Many chefs enjoy the challenge and will create excellent meals for you. You become a regular with a known diet they accommodate automatically.

For travel:

- Pack snacks: nuts, dried fruit, whole grain crackers
- Research restaurants before traveling
- Stay in accommodations with kitchen access if possible
- Grocery store runs: most grocery stores have fruit, vegetables, nuts, legumes

For cultural cuisine limitations, learn to cook your preferred cuisines plant based. Thai curry, Indian dal, Mexican beans, these are delicious when made plant based. When dining out, order closest to plant-based and adjust. Most cuisines have plant-forward expressions; they're sometimes just hidden on the menu.

Perspective Shift

Restaurant and travel challenges are logistical, not fundamental. They require planning and sometimes creativity, but they're solvable. You're not trapped. You're just playing a different game, one that requires intention rather than default. This builds mastery. Within weeks, you know which restaurants work, which cuisines are easiest, which snacks travel best. The challenge becomes routine.

Obstacle 8: Cravings and Temptation

UNDERSTANDING WHAT'S HAPPENING

You're doing well. Then someone brings your previous favorite food. Or you're stressed and suddenly crave something non-protocol. Or you're at an event and the pull toward indulgence feels irresistible.

Root causes:

- Habit (your brain expects certain foods at certain times)
- Stress or emotional discomfort (food is familiar comfort)
- Social situations (others are eating; peer influence)
- Nutrient deficiency (sometimes cravings signal missing nutrients)

Immediate Solution

- **Delay, don't deny.** When intense craving hits, drink water, take a walk, call your support person. Wait fifteen minutes. Cravings typically peak and pass.
- **Understand the craving.** Are you genuinely hungry or emotionally seeking comfort? If genuinely hungry, eat protocol-aligned food abundantly. If emotionally seeking comfort, address the emotion, call someone, go for a walk, journal rather than eating.

- **Replace the craving.** If you crave sweets, eat fruit or dates. If you crave salty, eat nuts or salted popcorn. If you crave rich/creamy, eat nut butter or tahini. Often, a protocol-aligned food satisfies the craving.

Deeper Solution

For habit-based cravings, after about four weeks, these largely resolve. Your taste buds are recalibrating. The intensity and frequency of cravings decrease dramatically. If you're past thirty days and still experiencing intense cravings, ensure you're not nutrient deficient (particularly iron, zinc, or B vitamins).

For stress-based eating, develop alternative coping mechanisms. When stressed, do you take a walk, call someone, journal, meditate, exercise? Practice these before stress hits, so they're available when stress arrives. Food becomes less appealing as a coping mechanism when better options are established.

For social eating pressure, eat something before the event so you're not hungry. Bring a dish to share (plant-based, so you know you can eat). Focus on socializing rather than eating. Stand away from food. Often, being full and focused on conversation removes the eating urge.

Perspective Shift

Cravings are normal, especially in the first thirty days. They're not failures. They're habit and chemistry recalibrating. By thirty to sixty days in, cravings largely resolve. What took months or years to become a habit takes weeks to become a new habit. When cravings do emerge (which is normal even after months), they're information: are you hungry, stressed, or habituated? Respond to the actual need, not the surface craving.

Obstacle 9: Work/Life Pressures

UNDERSTANDING WHAT'S HAPPENING

Work is intense. Family responsibilities are high. Stress is pervasive. In the midst of this, maintaining protocol adherence feels like one more thing, and it's easy to abandon.

Root causes:

- Limited time and energy for meal planning/prep
- Stress driving toward familiar comfort foods
- Mental fatigue reducing decision capacity
- Feeling like health needs are secondary to urgent demands

Immediate Solution

- **Simplify during high-stress periods.** Don't experiment with new recipes. Eat simple, repetitive meals: oatmeal for breakfast, salad for lunch, rice and beans for dinner. Consistency beats perfection during stress.
- **Batch cook when you can.** If stress permits, dedicate one to two hours on Sunday to preparing vegetables, grains, and legumes. Throughout the week, you're assembling rather than cooking.
- **Lower your bar temporarily.** During intense periods, maintaining 90 percent protocol adherence while managing stress is better than abandoning it entirely to reduce mental load. Give yourself permission to simplify and be less perfect.

Deeper Solution

For time pressure, meal prep isn't a luxury; it's a necessity. Block Sunday afternoon off for two to three hours. This investment saves you at least thirty minutes daily throughout the week. It's actually efficient, not an additional burden.

For stress-driven eating, recognize stress as an obstacle, not failure. During high-stress periods, protocol adherence becomes harder. Accept this. Maintain it anyway. The protocol actually helps stress (stable glucose = stable mood). Paradoxically, during stress, protocol adherence is most important and most challenging.

For decision fatigue, reduce decisions. Same breakfast daily. Same lunch formula. Same dinner structure. On Monday, you make one decision (which protein), and it's decided for the week. This reduces cognitive load dramatically.

Perspective Shift

Stress is when protocol adherence matters most. Your body is under pressure. It needs stable glucose, excellent nutrients, and optimal mitochondrial function to handle stress. Abandoning the protocol during stress is exactly backward. Embrace the protocol as stress management. Use it to stabilize yourself amidst chaos. By maintaining it despite stress, you prove its importance and deepen your commitment.

Obstacle 10: Family Resistance

UNDERSTANDING WHAT'S HAPPENING

Your family doesn't support this. They question your choices. They pressure you to return to previous eating. They don't understand. They're worried. They're resistant.

This is complex because it involves people you care about and your home environment.

Root causes:

- Fear (they're worried you're malnourished or hurting yourself)
- Cultural/family food traditions being challenged
- Implicit challenge to their own choices
- Lack of understanding about plant-based nutrition

Immediate Solution

- **Have a respectful conversation.** Explain you're doing this for your health. Share improvements in specific terms (better energy, better sleep, medical markers improved). Invite their questions. Don't be defensive.
- **Invite participation.** Invite family to try meals you're preparing. Let them experience delicious food. Allow them to see you thriving. Often, skepticism dissolves with direct experience.
- **Establish boundaries.** "I appreciate your concern, and I need to make this choice for my health. I'd love your support, but I understand if this is difficult. Either way, I'm continuing." Respectfully firm.

Deeper Solution

For worried family members, invite them to your health care provider appointments. Let them hear from a professional that this is safe and beneficial. Let them see your improved medical markers. Professional validation often reassures families more than your explanation alone.

For cultural/family food tradition challenges, adapt—don't reject—traditions. Learn to prepare family dishes plant based. Show that honoring tradition and honoring your health aren't mutually exclusive. Often, families discover they enjoy plant-based versions of familiar foods.

For implicit challenge to their choices, don't evangelize. Don't suggest others should adopt this protocol. Just live your own journey. Many people feel defensive when others make different choices it feels like judgment. Avoid that dynamic. "I'm doing this for me" is different from "You should do this too."

For family members who remain unsupportive, know that, ultimately, you are responsible for your health. You're not responsible for others' comfort with your choices. Some family members will come around. Some may take years. Some may never understand. Love them anyway. Maintain your boundaries anyway. Your health is not contingent on their approval.

Perspective Shift

Family resistance is real and worth acknowledging. It's also not your responsibility to resolve. You can invite understanding. You can share your journey. You can invite participation. But you cannot force acceptance. What you can do is live so visibly transformed in energy, health, and well-being that resistance gradually softens. People support what works. Your thriving is the most powerful argument for this protocol.

The Obstacle Mindset: Seeing Challenges as Evolution

As you navigate these obstacles, remember that obstacles aren't signs of failure. They're signs of real-world implementation.

Easy things don't require obstacles to navigate. They're already easy. The obstacles you're encountering hunger, social pressure, travel challenges, family resistance these are the *actual* real-world context of health restoration. Navigating them successfully isn't a bonus; it's the core practice of making this permanent.

Each obstacle you successfully navigate deepens your capability. Each challenge you overcome strengthens your commitment. Each person you respectfully hold boundaries with teaches you that your health is worth protecting. Each restaurant you learn to navigate builds your confidence.

By the time you've navigated multiple obstacles, you're not temporarily following a protocol. You're a person who has integrated health restoration into your actual life with its real pressures and real complexities.

This is mastery. This is permanence.

The obstacles don't disappear. But you develop such sophisticated navigation tools that they become routine rather than threatening.

Summary: Obstacles as Opportunities

OBSTACLE	ROOT CAUSE	IMMEDIATE RESPONSE	DEEPER SOLUTION
Persistent hunger	Insufficient calories/protein or habit-based hunger	Increase legumes, grains, nuts; track food	Adequate calories (1,800–2,500), proper meal composition
Persistent fatigue	Insufficient nutrition or excessive exercise	Increase calories; reduce exercise intensity	Track nutrients; ensure adequate iron, B12
Slow glucose improvement	Hidden refined carbs or nonadherence	Read labels meticulously; return to whole foods	100 percent adherence; underlying condition evaluation if needed

(continued)

OBSTACLE	ROOT CAUSE	IMMEDIATE RESPONSE	DEEPER SOLUTION
Digestive discomfort	Fiber increase or inadequate hydration	Hydrate extensively; chew thoroughly	Fermented foods; allow adaptation time; see provider if persistent
Inadequate weight loss	Muscle gain or calorie excess	Focus on body composition and how you feel	Track calories modestly; weight normalizes over time
Social pressure	People's fear and food as social/cultural practice	Set boundaries compassionately; find your people	Share results; lead by example; build community
Restaurant/travel challenges	Limited plant-based options available	Call ahead; know plant-friendly cuisines; eat before/after	Learn to cook preferred cuisines; build relationships with restaurants
Cravings	Habit, stress, or nutrient deficiency	Delay fifteen minutes; address actual need; replace with protocol-aligned food	Allow four to six weeks for habit recalibration; address stress management
Work/life pressure	Limited time and energy	Simplify meals; batch cook; lower perfection bar	Recognize stress periods as when protocol matters most
Family resistance	Fear, tradition challenge, or implicit judgment	Have respectful conversation; invite participation	Invite to appointments; adapt traditions; maintain boundaries

Each obstacle has a solution. Each solution reinforces your mastery. You're not following a protocol. You're becoming a person for whom health is integrated into every context of your life.

11

PERSONALIZATION: HONORING YOUR UNIQUE ENERGY SYSTEM

Introduction: The Protocol Is a Framework, Not a Prison

You've completed thirty days of protocol adherence. You've navigated obstacles. You've experienced your energy system restoration. You understand the ten principles. You know your medical markers have improved.

But you're wondering: *Is this exactly how I need to eat forever? Or can I adjust it to fit my life?*

This chapter gives you permission for what you've likely already intuited: the protocol is a framework, not a prison.

The ten principles are non-negotiable because they're aligned with your biology. Whole foods, plant-based, no refined carbs, no processed additives these aren't arbitrary restrictions. They're expressions of how your energy system is designed.

But how do you express those principles within your life? That's yours to personalize.

One person thrives on three meals daily. Another thrives on five smaller meals or intermittent fasting. One person eats 80 percent raw foods. Another eats mostly cooked foods. One person prefers carbohydrate-forward meals. Another prefers lower-carb, higher-legume meals. One person is an athlete requiring high calorie intake. Another is a grandmother maintaining stable energy for caregiving.

All of these people can honor the ten principles while personalizing their expression.

This chapter teaches you to create your own protocol, one that honors the principles while fitting your unique body, circumstances, preferences, and life. By the time you finish this chapter, you'll understand that protocol adherence isn't about rigid compliance. It's about intelligent personalization within a framework that works.

Let's build your protocol.

Part 1: The Personalization Framework

Personalizing means start with the standard protocol, observe your response for two to four weeks, identify what's working well, identify what could be adjusted, make small adjustments, and continue observing and refining.

Over four to week weeks, you emerge with YOUR protocol—one that honors the ten principles while fitting your unique energy system.

WEEK 1–2: STANDARD PROTOCOL

Follow the recommendations from Chapters 6–10 precisely. This is your baseline. You need baseline data to personalize intelligently.

WEEK 2–4: OBSERVATION

Track:

- Energy levels throughout the day
- Sleep quality
- Mental clarity
- Mood stability
- Digestive comfort
- Satiation at meals
- Physical performance
- Overall well-being

Write this down. You're creating data.

WEEK 4–5: ANALYSIS AND ADJUSTMENT

Ask yourself:

- What meals do I love? (Keep these.)
- What meals feel mediocre? (Consider adjusting.)
- How's my energy? (Optimal? Could it be higher? Could it be more stable?)
- How's my hunger? (Appropriate? Too high? Can you ignore hunger between meals?)
- How's my sleep? (Excellent? Could it be better?)
- What specific improvements would enhance my experience?

Make *one* or *two* small adjustments. Not radical changes. Small modifications. Examples:

- "I feel better with an extra meal, so I'll eat four smaller meals instead of three."

- "My energy is highest when I eat more grains and legumes and fewer raw vegetables, so I'll increase my intake of cooked foods."
- "I perform better in workouts with a carbohydrate meal pre-workout, so I'll add that into my timing."

WEEK 6–8: OBSERVATION OF ADJUSTMENT

Live with your adjustments for two to three weeks. Observe impact. Is energy better? Worse? The same? Make decisions based on data, not ideology.

WEEKS 8+: CONTINUED REFINEMENT

You now have *your* protocol. Continue observing. Make small adjustments as needed. Your protocol evolves as your life circumstances evolve.

Part 2: Personalization Areas

AREA 1: CARBOHYDRATE SENSITIVITY AND TOLERANCE

People have different carbohydrate tolerances. This varies based on:

- Insulin sensitivity (how efficiently cells respond to insulin)
- Activity level (athletes need more carbs)
- Metabolic rate
- Genetic factors

Observation questions:

- After eating carbohydrate-rich meals, do you feel energized or sluggish?
- Do you have afternoon energy crashes?
- How are your blood glucose readings?

High carbohydrate tolerance (most people):

- 45–65 percent of calories from carbohydrates
- Meals include vegetables + legumes/grains + fruit + nuts
- Example: Large salad + chickpeas + whole grain bread + fruit
- This is the standard protocol recommendation

Moderate carbohydrate tolerance:

- 40–50 percent of calories from carbohydrates
- Higher proportion of legumes relative to grains
- More nonstarchy vegetables, fewer starchy carbs
- Example: Vegetables + lentils + small portion of rice + nuts

Lower carbohydrate tolerance (some people, especially with PCOS):

- 30–40 percent of calories from carbohydrates
- Emphasis on vegetables, legumes, and nuts
- Minimal grain consumption
- Example: Large vegetable portion + beans + nuts, minimal grain

Important note: Even "lower carbohydrate" in plant-based context means legume/vegetable carbs, not processed carbs. You're not going ketogenic. You're just emphasizing vegetables and legumes over grains.

AREA 2: MEAL FREQUENCY

People's bodies operate optimally at different meal frequencies.

Observation questions:

- How do you feel with three meals daily?
- Do you get hungry between meals?
- Do you have stable energy or crashes?

Three meals daily (standard):

- Breakfast, lunch, dinner
- No snacks unless genuinely hungry
- Meals spaced approximately four to five hours apart
- Ideal for people with stable blood glucose, normal hunger patterns

Four to six smaller meals:

- Meals every two and a half to three hours
- Smaller portion size per meal
- May include snacks between meals
- Ideal for people with very active jobs, athletes, people with hypoglycemia history, very high metabolic rates

Intermittent fasting (IF):

- Eating window of six to eight hours, fasting window of sixteen to eighteen hours
- Example: Eating 12 p.m.–8 p.m., fasting 8 p.m.–12 p.m. the next day
- Two substantial meals or three smaller meals within eating window
- Ideal for people with good metabolic flexibility, no history of disordered eating, people who prefer fewer meal prep occasions

Note on IF: Intermittent fasting is compatible with plant-based protocol. However, ensure your eating window includes sufficient calories and nutrients. It's the quality of eating during the eating window that matters.

AREA 3: RAW VS. COOKED FOOD BALANCE

Raw foods have maximum enzyme content and heat-sensitive vitamins. Cooked foods are easier to digest and allow different nutrient absorption.

Observation questions:

- How do you feel with high raw food intake?
- Do you have digestive discomfort with lots of raw food?
- Do you perform better athletically with cooked foods?

High raw (50–80 percent raw):

- Emphasis on fresh vegetables and fruits in raw form
- Cooked legumes and grains still included (necessary for digestibility)
- Raw salads at most meals
- Ideal for people who digest raw foods easily, people sensitive to cooked food temperature, people with strong digestive systems

Balanced (30–50 percent raw):

- Mix of raw and cooked vegetables
- Raw fruit, raw nuts/seeds
- Cooked legumes, grains, and some cooked vegetables
- This is the standard protocol recommendation
- Ideal for most people

High cooked (20–30 percent raw):

- Most vegetables lightly cooked (steamed, roasted)
- Raw fruit maintained
- Raw nuts/seeds maintained
- Cooked legumes and grains
- Ideal for people with weak digestive systems, people recovering from illness, senior populations, people with digestive conditions (IBS, and so on)

AREA 4: FOOD PREFERENCES AND CULTURAL CONTEXT

Your protocol should include foods you genuinely enjoy and that honor your cultural identity.

Observation questions:

- What cuisines do you love?
- What are your favorite plant foods?
- What are your cultural food traditions?
- How can you adapt these plant-based?

Indian cuisine: Already largely plant-based friendly. Dal, chickpea curries, vegetable curries, rice, beans. You're not adapting much, just emphasizing the plant-based dishes.

Mediterranean cuisine: Naturally plant heavy. Legume dishes, abundant vegetables, olive oil—the only adjustment is moving away from extracted oils toward whole food fats.

Asian cuisines: Many Asian cuisines are predominantly plant-based. Tofu dishes, vegetable stir-fries, rice, and legume dishes. These align beautifully with the protocol.

Mexican cuisine: Beans are central. Tortillas, rice, vegetables, beans, salsa. These are already protocol-aligned. Emphasis on beans rather than meat.

African cuisines: Many African cuisines feature legumes, grains, and vegetables. Lentil stews, bean dishes, grain-based meals. These adapt beautifully.

Your protocol: Include cuisines you love. Adapt family recipes plant based. Make this personal and cultural, not generic.

AREA 5: ACTIVITY LEVEL AND ENERGY NEEDS

Physical activity affects energy and nutrient needs.

Observation questions:

- What's your activity level? (Sedentary, lightly active, very active, athlete)
- How do you feel with current calorie intake?
- Do you have energy for your desired activity?

Sedentary to lightly active:

- 1,800–2,200 calories daily (depending on body size)
- Three meals daily
- Standard protocol portions
- This is baseline for many people

Very active (regular exercise, physical job):

- 2,200–2,800 calories daily (depending on body size and activity intensity)
- Four to six meals daily to support energy needs

- Larger portions at meals
- Pre-workout carbohydrate meal (one to two hours before activity)
- Post-workout recovery meal (within thirty minutes after activity)

Athletes (intense training, competitive sports):

- 2,800–4,000+ calories daily (depending on body size, sport, training intensity)
- Multiple meals and snacks throughout day
- Timing of meals around training
- Higher emphasis on carbohydrates for fuel
- Adequate protein for recovery (1.2–2 g per kg bodyweight)

Your protocol: Adjust portions and meal frequency based on your activity level. More activity requires more fuel. Ensure you're eating enough to support your activity without excessive surplus.

AREA 6: AGE-RELATED CONSIDERATIONS

Nutritional needs and optimal approaches vary by life stage.

Younger adults (twenties to forties):

- High metabolic flexibility
- Can tolerate varied eating patterns
- Often very active
- Standard protocol works well for most

Midlife adults (forties to sixties):

- Metabolism often slowing
- May have beginning metabolic markers requiring attention
- Often juggling multiple responsibilities
- May benefit from more structured meal planning

Older adults (sixties and over):

- Digestive capacity may be reduced (smaller, more frequent meals preferable)
- Protein needs may be higher (1.0–1.2 g per kg bodyweight)
- Chewing capacity may be reduced (softer foods preferable)
- More emphasis on cooked foods often helpful
- Special attention to nutrient absorption (B12, iron, calcium particularly important)

Your age consideration: Adjust based on your life stage. Older adults may benefit from smaller, more frequent meals with more cooked foods. Younger, very active adults may thrive on larger meals and higher carbohydrate intake.

AREA 7: HEALTH CONDITION CONSIDERATIONS

Specific health conditions may benefit from personalized protocol adjustments.

Type 2 Diabetes:

- May benefit from lower carbohydrate load within plant-based framework
- Emphasis on legumes and vegetables over grains
- Monitor blood glucose closely; work with health care provider

PCOS (polycystic ovary syndrome):

- Insulin resistance common; lower carbohydrate approach often beneficial
- Higher protein from legumes and nuts
- Consistent meal timing (helps hormone regulation)

Hypertension:

- Emphasis on potassium-rich foods (vegetables, legumes, fruit)
- Limited sodium (sea salt minimal)
- Often improves rapidly on protocol

Arthritis/joint pain:

- High plant-based foods reduce inflammation
- May benefit from emphasis on anti-inflammatory foods (turmeric, ginger, leafy greens)
- Omega-3 sources (flax, chia, walnuts) beneficial

IBS/digestive conditions:

- May require higher emphasis on cooked foods
- Soluble fiber (oatmeal, fruit) may be better tolerated than insoluble
- Smaller, more frequent meals often helpful
- Work with health care provider

Your health condition: If you have a specific health condition, research plant-based approaches to it. Work with your health care provider. Make personalized adjustments.

AREA 8: LIFE CIRCUMSTANCE CONSIDERATIONS

Your life circumstances affect what's sustainable.

High stress periods:

- Simplify meals (same breakfast, lunch, dinner daily)
- Batch cooking becomes more important
- Slightly lower expectations for variety

- Maintenance is success during stress

Travel/nomadic lifestyle:

- Portable, shelf-stable foods become important (nuts, dried fruit, whole grain crackers)
- Restaurant navigation skills essential
- Flexibility becomes more important
- Perfect adherence less important than reasonable approximation

Limited budget:

- Dried beans and lentils are cheapest protein
- Seasonal, local vegetables are most economical
- Grains in bulk are inexpensive
- Focus on these fundamentals
- Special foods (nuts, supplements) are optional

Family with different diets:

- Prepare core ingredients family can customize
- Example: Cooked rice and beans as base; family adds different sides/proteins
- Your meal can be plant-based; others can add animal products if they choose
- Reduces burden of cooking multiple separate meals

Your life circumstances: Design a protocol that works within your actual life, not some idealized version. A protocol you actually maintain is infinitely better than a perfect protocol you abandon.

Part 3: Special Populations

PREGNANT AND BREASTFEEDING WOMEN

Nutritional considerations:

- Increased calorie needs (300+ calories daily during pregnancy, 500 during breastfeeding)
- Increased protein needs (71 g daily during pregnancy)
- Critical nutrients: iron, calcium, B12, omega-3s, iodine
- Work closely with health care provider
- Consider supplementation: B12, iron, omega-3s, iodine (all appropriate for plant-based pregnancy)

Practical approach:

- Eat three substantial meals plus one to two snacks daily
- Include protein source at each meal (legumes, nuts, seeds)
- Calcium-rich foods (leafy greens, fortified plant milk, tahini)
- Iron-rich foods (legumes, grains, dark leafy greens) with vitamin C for absorption
- Adequate calories for healthy weight gain

CHILDREN AND ADOLESCENTS

Nutritional considerations:

- Growing bodies need adequate protein, calories, and specific nutrients
- Young children: smaller, more frequent meals
- Adolescents: high calorie and protein needs (especially if active)
- Critical nutrients: iron, B12, calcium, iodine
- Work with pediatrician familiar with plant-based nutrition

Practical approach:

- Include protein at each meal and snack
- Calcium-rich foods daily (dark leafy greens, fortified plant milk, tahini)
- B12 supplementation or fortified foods essential
- Adequate calories for growth
- Variety of foods to ensure micronutrient diversity

ATHLETES

Nutritional considerations:

- High calorie needs (2,800–4,000+ daily)
- High protein needs (1.2–2 g/kg bodyweight)
- Carbohydrate timing around workouts
- Hydration and electrolyte needs
- Work with sports nutritionist familiar with plant-based diet

Practical approach:

- Multiple meals and snacks throughout day
- Carbohydrate meal two to three hours before workout
- Recovery meal (carbs + protein) within thirty minutes post-workout
- Adequate total protein from legumes, nuts, seeds, whole grains
- Adequate calories to support training without energy deficit

SENIORS (SIXTY-FIVE AND OVER)

Nutritional considerations:

- Potentially reduced digestive capacity
- Potentially reduced nutrient absorption
- Higher protein needs (1.0–1.2g/ kg bodyweight)
- Critical nutrients: B12, iron, calcium, vitamin D, omega-3s
- Medication interactions (work with pharmacist)

Practical approach:

- Smaller, more frequent meals (four to five daily)
- Softer foods if chewing difficult
- More emphasis on cooked foods than raw
- Nutrient-dense foods (vegetables, legumes, nuts, seeds, whole grains)
- B12 supplementation or fortified foods essential
- Regular health monitoring with health care provider

PEOPLE WITH LIMITED INCOME

Nutritional considerations:

- Budget constraints are real
- Still can eat fully protocol-aligned on limited budget
- Focus on inexpensive staples

Practical approach:

- Dried beans and lentils (pennies per serving)
- Seasonal vegetables (cheaper than out-of-season)
- Grains in bulk (rice, oats, barley)
- Canned vegetables if fresh unavailable
- Canned beans if dried beans not accessible
- Minimal focus on "special" foods (nuts, supplements, specialty items)
- This protocol is actually the most economical real-food diet available

Part 4: The Personalization Permission

Here's what you need to understand: You have permission to personalize.

You've proven you can follow the protocol. You've experienced its benefits. You understand the principles. Now you have permission to make this yours.

Some people thrive with strict adherence to the standard protocol. That's perfect. Continue exactly as outlined.

Others thrive with modifications, such as higher raw or lower raw. More meals or fewer meals. Higher carb or lower carb. With activity or without. Whatever works for your body, within the framework of the ten principles.

This personalization isn't a betrayal of the protocol. It's the ultimate expression of it taking the scientifically sound, biologically aligned framework and expressing it in a way that fits your unique energy system.

Your protocol might look different than your neighbor's protocol, and that's perfect. You're both honoring the ten principles. You're both restoring your energy systems. You're both healing. The specific expression is yours.

Part 5: Section 2 Completion—Your Transformation

Let's pause and acknowledge what you've accomplished.

Thirty days ago, you:

- Were experiencing dysregulated energy (crashes, fatigue, unstable mood)
- Had medical markers indicating energy system dysfunction
- Didn't know if this was possible for you

Today, you:

- Have stable, abundant energy throughout your day
- Have medical markers showing restoration
- Have proven to yourself that your body can heal
- Have navigated real-world obstacles
- Have created a personalized protocol that works for your unique life
- Know that this is permanent

This is a profound transformation. Not because you're following someone else's rules. But because you've fundamentally restored your energy system.

Section 2 has taught you:

- **Why** this protocol works (philosophy + science of energy restoration)
- **How** to implement it (practical pathway from understanding to action)
- **What to expect** (thirty-day timeline with physiological detail)
- **How to measure it** (medical markers validating what you feel)
- **How to troubleshoot it** (real-world obstacles with solutions)
- **How to sustain it** (personalized expression that fits your life)

You now understand energy restoration at the deepest level. Not intellectually alone, but experientially. You've lived it. You've measured it. You've adjusted it. You've made it yours.

Part 6: Bridging to Section 3

Section 3 shifts focus from general energy restoration to disease-specific reversal.

You've proven that aligned nutrition restores your energy system. Now we explore: *What disease reversal becomes possible when your energy system is fully restored?*

Section 3 will address:

- Heart disease reversal (Chapter 12)
- Weight normalization (Chapter 13)
- Mental health and cognitive function (Chapter 14)
- Disease prevention and comprehensive wellness (Chapter 15)

These aren't separate from what you've learned. They're expressions of it. When your energy system is restored, your body naturally tends toward the reversal of conditions that required dysregulated energy to maintain.

Your personal health condition whether it's heart disease, weight dysregulation, depression, cognitive decline, or disease prevention becomes the lens through which you understand your continued restoration.

By the end of Section 3, you'll understand not just how to restore energy generally, but how to apply that restoration specifically to whatever health challenge you're addressing.

The Personalized Protocol Template

You will find a template for creating your own written protocol on the following page—your personalized expression of the ten principles.

MY ENERGY RESTORATION PROTOCOL

NAME: [Your name]   **DATE STARTED:** [Date]

BASELINE ENERGY LEVEL: [1–10]

MY PERSONALIZED APPROACH:

Meal frequency: [three meals / four to five meals / intermittent fasting / other]

Raw vs. cooked balance: [percent raw, percent cooked]

Carbohydrate emphasis: [Higher carb (grains emphasis) / Moderate / Lower carb (legume/vegetable emphasis)]

Favorite cuisines: [Your favorite plant-based cuisines]

Key foods I love: [Specific vegetables, legumes, grains, nuts, seeds you particularly enjoy]

Activity level: [Sedentary / Lightly active / Very active / Athlete]

Daily calorie target: [Based on your activity level]

Special considerations: [Health conditions, life circumstances, age-related factors, budget considerations]

MY TYPICAL DAY:

Breakfast: [Your typical breakfast]

Lunch: [Your typical lunch]

Dinner: [Your typical dinner]

Snacks (if applicable): [Your typical snacks]

HOW I FEEL ON THIS PROTOCOL:

Energy: [1–10]

Sleep: [Quality and duration]

Mental clarity: [1–10]

Mood: [1–10]

Physical symptoms: [Any relevant improvements]

Adjustments I've made from standard protocol: [Describe what you've personalized]

Why these adjustments work for me: [Explain your rationale]

Write this out. Make it real. This is *your* protocol. This is your personalized expression of the ten principles. This is your energy restoration, customized to your unique life.

Final Reflection: From Protocol to Lifestyle

The journey from dysregulated energy to restored energy to personalized sustainability is profound.

You didn't just change what you eat. You changed how your energy system functions. You didn't just follow a diet. You aligned your body with its biological design. You didn't just treat symptoms. You restored the foundation that allows your body to express its inherent capacity for health.

And you did it in a way that fits your life, your preferences, your culture, your activity level, your circumstances, your unique energy system.

This is mastery. This is personalization. This is yours.

The protocol was the framework. But you, your intelligence, your preferences, your unique biology, you're the artist. The framework is there. The principles are non-negotiable. But how do you express them? That's your masterpiece.

My Transformation Journey

From Decision Through Achievement to Thriving—The Proof of What Energy Restoration Creates in Real Life

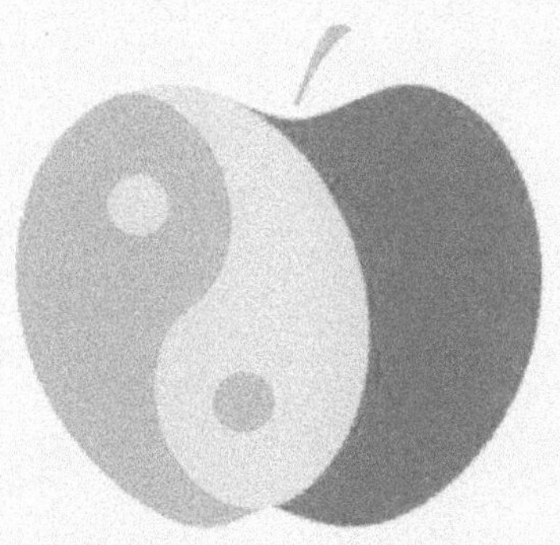

12

THE BEGINNING

December 6, 2009, The Decision That Changed Everything

OPENING: NOT PERFECTION, BUT A DECISION

This is not a story about a man who became perfect overnight. This is *my* story. On December 6, 2009, at age fifty, I made the decision "If it's not made by Mother Nature, it's not going on my plate."

That decision was imperfect from the start. That decision was messy. That decision evolved year after year. And that decision sustained for sixteen years with commitment, flexibility, and continuous evolution reversed the trajectory of a life that had been heading toward the complications of Type 2 diabetes.

THE STARTING POINT: AGE FIFTY, TYPE 2 PREDIABETES

In 2004, five years before this story began, Type 2 prediabetes had been diagnosed. My medical records showed it clearly: elevated glucose, rising inflammation markers, the beginning of a path that could lead to kidney disease, nerve damage, heart disease, blindness.

The statistics were clear that most people with Type 2 prediabetes develop serious complications within ten to fifteen years. It was not a matter of if. It was a matter of when.

By 2009, at age fifty, the trajectory seemed set. Medications managed symptoms. Doctors provided standard advice. Life proceeded as expected for someone with Type 2 diabetes.

But something in me was asking a different question.

THE CATALYST: A BROTHER-IN-LAW'S CHALLENGE

My transformation didn't begin with a dramatic health crisis or a desperate medical ultimatum. It began on December 6, 2009, during my mother's birthday celebration.

My brother-in-law made a simple challenge: "Don't wait until New Year's Day to start. Start today."

I made the decision: "Today, I commit to eating only foods made by Mother Nature. No processed foods. No industry-made products. Only what nature provides."

December 6, 2009. Age fifty. Type 2 prediabetes diagnosed. No medications ready to be discontinued. No dramatic life circumstances forcing change. Just a decision that changed everything.

The Reality: Not Perfect from Day 1

Here's the truth that most health stories don't tell: it wasn't perfect.

Early 2010 (first months):

- Breakfast: Granola bars (still processed, but I perceived them as "healthy")
- Dinner: Ragu pasta sauce mixed with vegetables (processed sauce, but I was moving away from cooked meals)
- Snacks: A mix of processed and whole foods
- Mindset: "I'm doing plant-based raw food, but I haven't figured out all the details yet."

I was making a commitment to a direction (plant-based, raw foods, no industry products) while still living in the world where processed foods were the default.

Was this "perfect raw food"? No.

Was this "100 percent compliant with the protocol"? No.

Was this the decision point that changed everything? *Yes*.

The Principle That Enabled Sixteen Years: Raw First—Not Perfection

What emerged from those early months wasn't a rigid set of rules. What emerged was a principle: Raw first—not perfection.

This principle meant:

- **Raw first:** When faced with a choice, I chose the rawest, least processed option available.
- **Not perfection:** If the perfect raw option wasn't available, I chose the best available option.
- **Progress over purity:** The direction matters more than the perfection of each individual choice
- **Sustainability over strictness:** A flexible approach I could maintain for over sixteen years beats a perfect approach I would quit after six months.

Year 1: Awareness and Transition (2010)

CREATING PERSONAL RULES—AGE FIFTY TO FIFTY-ONE

THE FIRST YEAR OF EVOLUTION—AGE FIFTY TO FIFTY-ONE

The first year was about awareness.

What changed:

- Granola bars: Removed. I replaced them with raw nuts, seeds, and whole fruits. Simple swap. Processed carbohydrates + added sugars → whole nuts + natural sweetness.
- Ragu pasta sauce: Recognized as processed. What could replace it? Fresh tomatoes blended into sauce. Then I eliminated pasta sauce entirely and ate raw vegetables in homemade salsa or chutney vinegar instead.
- Subtle observation: How did my body respond to different foods?

This wasn't intellectual analysis. It was a lived experience. When I replaced granola bars with raw almonds, walnuts, and dates, my energy didn't crash by 10 a.m. The typical midmorning fatigue didn't appear. My concentration improved.

When I switched lunch from processed meats to vegetables and nuts, I felt more satisfied. When I replaced cooked pasta with raw vegetables at dinner, my digestion improved noticeably.

My body was providing feedback. The protocol wasn't abstract theory. It felt experience.

My doctors said, "Your glucose levels are improving. Keep going."

Not "You're perfect." But, "You're heading in the right direction. Keep going."

Year 2: Deepening the Commitment (2011)

CREATING PERSONAL RULES—AGE FIFTY-ONE TO FIFTY-TWO

By Year 2, a pattern had emerged. What foods supported my energy? What foods created fatigue? What choices led to better sleep, clearer thinking, more sustained energy?

My commitment deepened. But it wasn't imposed from outside. It came from my lived experience of what my body responded to.

I had a key realization that I don't need to follow someone else's rules. I need to discover *my* rules based on how *my* body responds.

This was liberating. This was personal. This was sustainable.

What changed:

- I eliminated more processed oils.
- I replaced processed snacks with whole foods.

- I created personal meal patterns based on energy response.
- I developed intuition about what supported my vitality.

My medical markers were changing. My HbA1C is improving. Liver function (ALT) improving. Blood pressure is stable. Energy is increasing.

The doctors said, "Excellent progress. Keep up what you're doing."

Years 3–16: Continuous Evolution (2012–2025)

THE LONG GAME OF EVOLUTION—AGES FIFTY-TWO TO SIXTY-SIX

What happened over the next thirteen years wasn't dramatic crisis-to-recovery. It was steady, continuous evolution.

During Year 3, I eliminated another category of processed foods. By Year 5, I discovered that certain food combinations supported better energy. In Year 7, I refined meal timing. In Year 10, I deepened my understanding of which raw foods supported athletic performance. And sixteen years in, I'm still discovering refinements, still evolving.

The pattern:

- No "I'm done and perfect" moment
- No "I've arrived and can relax"
- Only continuous awareness, continuous choice, continuous evolution

Each year brought:

- Better energy
- Improved athletic performance
- More refined understanding
- Deeper alignment with the protocol
- Stronger intuition about what supported my vitality

The Real Transformation: Energy as the Guide

Here's what nobody in the medical system was tracking: energy.

Doctors tracked:

- HbA1C levels
- Glucose readings
- Cholesterol panels
- Liver enzymes

I tracked:

- How I felt waking up
- My energy levels throughout the day
- My recovery from exercise
- My mental clarity
- My sleep quality
- My capacity for the life I wanted to live

The real transformation wasn't in the medical markers (though they improved dramatically). The real transformation was in my lived experience.

From 2009 to 2025:

- Energy: From baseline fatigue to sustained, abundant energy
- Capacity: From managing disease to training for marathons
- Vitality: From accepting age-related decline to thriving at sixty-six years young
- Freedom: From disease management to optimal living

The medical data validated what was already known through living: *the protocol works because my body responds to what it actually needs.*

The Critical Decade: Consistency Proves the Point

You may be wondering why sixteen years matter? One year of good health is a novelty. Five years is a pattern. Ten years is proof. Sixteen years is undeniable.

In Year 5, you think, "Maybe this is just a temporary improvement." By Year 10, "This is working, but will it last?" And then, when you get to Year 16, you think, "This is how health works. This is sustainable. This is my life."

Medical reality at Year 16:

- Type 2 Diabetes: Controlled without medications
- Diabetic complications: Zero (extremely rare)
- Athletic performance: Seven marathons completed, training for the eighth
- Health markers: All optimal
- Vital signs: Better than average forty year old
- Energy: Abundant and sustainable

Most diabetics develop serious complications within ten to fifteen years. I developed *none*, while completing marathons and maintaining elite athletic performance.

The protocol didn't just manage my disease. It reversed my trajectory. It prevented complications. It enabled optimal aging.

The Doctor's Perspective

Throughout sixteen years, one message remained consistent from my health care providers: *keep going.*

Not because I was perfect. Not because I was 100 percent compliant with some ideal protocol. But because:

- My energy markers improved
- My medical markers improved
- My athletic performance improved
- Zero complications emerged
- I didn't need medications
- My health trajectory reversed

Doctors see the results. Results speak louder than opinions. My doctors say, "Keep up what you're doing."

What This Teaches

This story teaches something critical that most health transformations don't demonstrate: You don't need perfection to create profound transformation.

You need:

1. **A clear direction:** "Toward whole foods, away from processed foods."
2. **Personal commitment:** "I'm doing this for my health."
3. **Flexibility:** "I'll evolve, adjust, and create *my own* rules."
4. **Energy awareness:** "I'll listen to how my body responds."
5. **Patience:** "This is a sixteen-year journey, not a sixteen-week fix."
6. **Consistency:** "I show up every day, even if imperfectly."

The result of sixteen years of this approach:

- Type 2 diabetes managed without medications
- Zero diabetic complications (extremely rare)
- Athletic performance at elite level
- Sustained energy and vitality
- Optimal health markers
- Freedom from disease trajectory

The Point

My story is not about reaching perfection on December 6, 2009.

My story is about making a decision on December 6, 2009, and then showing up, day after day, year after year, with flexibility, evolution, and commitment to a principle: Raw first—not perfection.

That decision, sustained for sixteen years, reversed the expected trajectory of Type 2 diabetes. It prevented complications that should have emerged. It enabled athletic performance that defies typical aging. It created a life of vitality and freedom.

Not because of perfection. Because of commitment. Because of evolution. Because of listening to my body. Because of sixteen years of showing up.

This is what sustained transformation looks like.

Looking Forward

My story of transformation doesn't end at year sixteen. It continues.

Energy guides my way. The protocol evolves. The principle remains: Raw first—not perfection.

At sixty-six years young, training for my eighth marathon, with optimal health markers and zero diabetic complications, my journey continues.

Not as someone who has arrived at perfection. But as someone who made a decision sixteen years ago, showed up every day with flexibility and commitment, and discovered that my body knows exactly what to do when given what it actually needs.

The Invitation

If you read this story thinking, "I could never be that perfect. I could never give up all processed foods. I could never be that committed," then you've misunderstood my story.

My story is not about perfection. It's about direction. It's about listening to your body. It's about creating *your own* rules based on how *your* body responds. It's about the principle: Raw first—not perfection.

You don't need to start perfect. You need to start. You need to evolve. You need to listen. You need to show up, imperfectly, for sixteen years.

That's my story.

That's my transformation.

That's what's possible.

13

YEAR-BY-YEAR EVOLUTION

How Energy Restoration Becomes Life: My Sixteen-Year Journey (2009–2025)

THE POWER OF CONSISTENCY

Transformation doesn't happen in a moment. It happens in moments.

One moment deciding to eat differently. One moment choosing a raw vegetable over processed food. One moment feeling my energy increase. One moment noticing better sleep. One moment running a little faster than yesterday.

Accumulated across sixteen years, these moments became my life.

This chapter follows my actual progression: not a dramatic before-and-after, but a real evolution. Year by year. Refinement by refinement. Choice by choice. Energy is increasing. Capacity growing. My body responded to what it was finally given.

Years 1–2: Foundation And Awareness (2009–2011)

AGES FIFTY-ONE TO FIFTY-TWO: CREATING THE FOUNDATION

The First Transition (2009–2010)

Day 1: December 6, 2009. The decision was made. But what did that mean, practically?

My breakfast changed first, from granola bars to raw almonds, walnuts, and dates. A simple swap. Processed carbohydrates and added sugars to whole nuts and natural sweetness.

What happened:

- My energy at breakfast didn't crash by 10 a.m. The typical midmorning fatigue didn't appear. My concentration improved.

- At lunch, I removed processed cooked food. I replaced them with fruits, nuts, and seeds. More filling. More sustaining. My energy stayed stable.
- At dinner, I recognized the Ragu pasta sauce for what it was: highly processed, laden with additives, salt, modified ingredients. What replaced it? Fresh tomatoes blended homemade salsa, chutney, vinegar with raw vegetables. Then I eliminated pasta sauce entirely. Raw vegetables became my main course.

This wasn't intellectual decision-making. It was an observation: "When I eat this, I feel better. When I eat that, I feel worse."

Medical markers (2010):

- HbA1C: Improving
- Liver function (ALT): Showing decline in inflammation
- Energy: Noticeably increased
- My doctor's comment: "Whatever you're doing, keep going."

I had a personal discovery that my body responds immediately to better nutrition. Energy is the feedback system.

Year 2: Deepening (2010–2011)

By Year 2, the pattern was clear: foods close to nature supported my energy. Processed foods depleted it.

Key discoveries:

- Refined carbohydrates: Created energy spikes and crashes. I eliminated them.
- Extracted oils: Created sluggishness and inflammation. I replaced them with whole nuts and seeds.
- Animal products: Not part of my protocol from the beginning, but processed versions were especially avoided.
- Whole fruits and vegetables: Sustained my energy, cleared my thinking, improved my sleep.

The critical shift: From following rules to creating my own personal rules. I asked myself, "What energizes *me*? What drains *me*? What supports *my* body's needs?"

The answers weren't the same as generic health advice. They were personal to me.

Personal rules I created:

- Breakfast: Raw fruits, nuts, seeds (or skip breakfast if not hungry)
- Lunch: Abundant fruits

- Dinner: Raw vegetables as primary, whole foods as complementary
- Snacks: Nuts, seeds, whole fruits
- Never: Processed cooked foods, extracted oils, refined ingredients

These weren't rigid rules. They were principles. Flexible enough to adapt to circumstances, firm enough to guide my decisions.

Medical markers (2011):

- HbA1C: 6.3–6.7 percent range (excellent for diabetic management)
- Liver function: Continuing to improve
- Blood pressure: Stable and healthy
- Triglycerides: Normalized
- Energy: Sustained throughout my day

Athletic beginning: I started thinking about movement. Running seemed possible. My energy supported it.

What my doctors said: "Your metabolic markers are excellent. Whatever lifestyle changes you've made are working. Keep it up."

Years 3–5: Deepening and Performance (2011–2014)

AGES FIFTY-TWO TO FIFTY-FOUR: ATHLETIC FOUNDATION BUILT

Running Begins (2011–2012)

By Year 3, energy was no longer a question for me. It was abundant. My body felt capable. Why not test it?

I began running. Not competitively. Not with grand ambitions. Just "can my body run?"

The answer was yes. More than that, my body thrived with movement.

Discovery: energy and movement reinforce each other.

- Better nutrition → More energy for exercise
- Exercise → My body demands better nutrition to recover
- The cycle reinforces both directions

My First Marathon (2009, Age Fifty)

I completed it. My body could do this.

But here's what's important: This wasn't an athlete's body doing what athletes do. This was a fifty-two-year-old person with Type 2 diabetes, previously living a sedentary lifestyle, discovering that my body responds to proper support.

Medical markers (2012–2013):

- HbA1C: Remained excellent (6.3–6.7 percent)
- Resting heart rate: Decreased (athletic adaptation beginning)
- Cholesterol panels: Excellent ratios
- Inflammation markers: Consistently improved

Years 4 and 5: Refinement (2013–2014)

I wasn't obsessing about nutrition or training. But I was observing.

What foods supported my marathon training? What meal timing supported my energy and recovery? What choices led to better sleep after long runs?

Through observation, my protocol refined itself.

Emerging understanding:

- Timing matters: When I eat affects my energy availability.
- Quantity matters: More training meant I needed to pay attention to adequate calories.
- Quality matters: Processed foods hindered my recovery; whole foods supported it.
- Rest matters: The protocol works best with adequate sleep and recovery.

By year five (2014, Age fifty-four):

- I completed three marathons
- My athletic performance was improving (faster times, quicker recovery)
- My energy was abundant
- I took no medications for diabetes
- My medical markers were all optimal

What was different: The protocol wasn't something I was "doing." It was becoming automatic. My body was used to whole foods. Processed foods felt wrong to me. The energy of my system was stabilized and thriving.

Years 6–10: Optimization and Excellence (2014–2019)

AGES FIFTY-FOUR TO FIFTY-NINE: PEAK ATHLETIC INTEGRATION

Systematic Refinement (2014–2016)

By Year 6, I wasn't learning basic principles. I was optimizing.

What had worked for marathons one through three? What could I refine for marathons four through five?

Discoveries in these years:

- Micronutrient awareness: I noticed which whole foods supported my best performance
- Meal timing optimization: I learned when to eat before/after training for best recovery
- Personal energy tracking: I understood my personal cycles and needs
- Injury prevention: Better nutrition meant faster healing, better injury prevention

My marathons four to five (2015–2017):

- Performance: My running times continued to improve (remarkable for a man in his fifties)
- Recovery: Faster recovery, less soreness
- Consistency: My training volume increased without injury

Medical Milestone (2016–2017, Ages Fifty-Six to Fifty-Seven)

My medical data showed something rare: a person with Type 2 diabetes running marathons, taking *no* medications, with *zero* complications.

Kidney function—perfect. Eyes—no diabetic damage. Feet—no neuropathy. Heart—running marathons.

This isn't supposed to happen. Most diabetics develop serious complications. I was doing the opposite, I was thriving athletically while managing my diabetes through the protocol alone.

Years 7–10 (2017–2019)

The protocol had become completely automatic. I wasn't making conscious choices anymore. My body knew what it needed. My choices were intuitive.

What changed:

- Conscious effort → Automatic habit
- "Following the protocol" → "Living the protocol"
- Thinking about food choices → Making choices naturally

COVID Impact (2020–2022)

A major disruption: the COVID-19 pandemic and lockdowns.

What happened: My running was disrupted. My physical activity decreased. The protocol worked for nutrition, but movement was compromised.

Real observation: Even with an optimal raw food diet, *movement* is essential. When my movement decreased during lockdown, my metabolic markers (especially triglycerides) spiked temporarily.

What this taught me: The protocol isn't just food. Food + movement + consistency = optimal health.

Years 11–16: Mastery and Sustained Vitality (2019–2025)

AGES FIFTY-NINE TO SIXTY-SIX: THRIVING AT ADVANCED AGE

Post-COVID Recovery and Continued Evolution (2022–2025)

When lockdowns ended and I resumed training, my body returned to optimal quickly. My triglycerides normalized. My athletic performance returned. The foundation was still there.

This period demonstrated something crucial: the protocol creates resilience.

When disrupted, my body recovered quickly. When I returned to the protocol, my vitality returned. My sixteen-year investment had created a body capable of thriving.

My Current State (2025, Age Sixty-Six Years Young)

My athletic performance:

- Seven marathons completed (Ages fifty to sixty-six)
- Currently training for my eighth marathon
- My running times are competitive with people decades younger
- My resting heart rate: 61 bpm (elite athlete range)

My medical markers (most recent, 2025):

- HbA1C: 5.9 percent (better than most people without diabetes)
- Blood pressure: 133/68 (optimal)
- Resting pulse: 61 bpm (athletic)
- BMI: 22.74 (ideal)
- Weight: 140 pounds at 5'6" (lean athletic build)
- Triglycerides: 100 mg/dL (excellent, recovered from COVID spike)
- Liver function (ALT): 21 (optimal, half of my baseline)
- Kidney function: Perfect, improving over time
- Diabetic complications: Zero

What's remarkable is that by every marker, I am healthier, stronger, more vital at sixty-six years young than most people at forty-five.

How My Energy Changed: The Real Progression

Medical markers are important validation. But the real story is my energy.

Year 1 (2009–2010):

- Energy: Increased from my baseline fatigue
- Experience: "I feel better in the mornings."
- Capacity: "I can do more than I thought."

Year 3 (2011–2012):

- Energy: Sustained throughout my day
- Experience: "I don't need caffeine or energy drinks."
- Capacity: "I can run a marathon."

Year 5 (2013–2014):

- Energy: Abundant and reliable
- Experience: "I have energy for everything I want to do."
- Capacity: "Running is becoming natural."

Year 10 (2018–2019):

- Energy: Stable, high, automatic
- Experience: "I don't think about energy. It's just there."
- Capacity: "Training feels good. Recovery is easy."

Year 16 (2024–2025):

- Energy: Abundant at sixty-six years young
- Experience: "I have more energy now than at fifty."
- Capacity: "Training for my eighth marathon feels achievable."

This is what energy restoration looks like—from depleted to abundant. From managed to thriving.

How My Protocol Evolved: Not Fixed, But Living

The protocol wasn't imposed from outside. It evolved from inside my own experience.

- **Year 1–2:** Basic elimination (I removed processed foods)
- **Year 3–5:** Intentional addition (I discovered which whole foods support me best)
- **Year 6–10:** Optimization (I fine-tuned timing, ratios, my personal preferences)
- **Year 11–16:** Mastery (I live it automatically, continue subtle refinement)

MY PERSONAL RULES AT EACH STAGE

Years 1–2 rules:

- No processed foods
- Eat whole plant foods
- Notice how my body responds

Years 3–5 rules:

- Emphasize foods that support my training
- Eat adequate nutrition for my athletic demands
- Continue eliminating foods that don't serve me

Years 6–10 rules:

- Optimize my meal timing around training
- Balance my macronutrients for sustained energy
- Maintain consistency while allowing flexibility

Years 11–16 rules:

- Trust my body's signals
- Maintain what works
- Continue evolving based on my life circumstances

The key principle through all these years is "raw first, not perfection."

At every stage, my goal wasn't perfection. It was direction. It was listening. It was progress.

WHAT DIDN'T CHANGE

Throughout sixteen years, several things remained constant for me:

- **My core commitment:** Raw foods made by nature, not processed foods made by industry.
- **My energy awareness:** I paid attention to how my body responds.
- **My doctor partnership:** I worked *with* health care providers, not against them.
- **My flexibility:** I created my own rules, not following rigid dogma.
- **My consistency:** I showed up every day, year after year.

WHAT CHANGED PROFOUNDLY

- **My energy:** From depleted to abundant
- **My capacity:** From limited to athletic excellence
- **My health:** From disease trajectory to optimal health

- **My freedom:** From disease management to thriving
- **My understanding:** From following rules to trusting my body

THE POWER OF SIXTEEN YEARS

My thinking evolved over time. In one year, I thought, "Maybe this is working." Five years in, I thought, "This works, but will it last?" Ten years in, I thought, "This is clearly working." And now sixteen years in, I think, "This is how health works."

By Year 16:

- I take no medications for Type 2 diabetes
- I have zero diabetic complications (extraordinarily rare)
- My athletic performance is at elite level
- All my health markers are optimal
- My energy is abundant
- My life is thriving

This is what sustained transformation looks like.

Not a dramatic before and after. But a real progression. Year after year. Choice after choice. My energy is increasing. My capacity is growing. My life is expanding.

The Real Teaching

This progression teaches something profound: I didn't transform overnight. I transformed through consistent, imperfect, evolving commitment to a principle.

The principle: Raw first, not perfection.

My commitment: Show up every day, even imperfectly.

My result: After sixteen years, my life is completely transformed.

Looking at My Data (Without Obsessing Over It)

Here's the reality: I wasn't obsessing over metrics. But my metrics validate my lived experience.

- **2004 (Starting point):** Type 2 diabetes diagnosed, inflammation high
- **2009 (Protocol begins):** Still Type 2 diabetes, beginning my protocol
- **2015 (five years in):** Type 2 diabetes controlled, three marathons completed
- **2020 (ten years in):** Type 2 diabetes controlled, five marathons completed, no complications
- **2025 (sixteen years in):** Type 2 diabetes controlled, seven marathons, zero complications, health markers of someone decades younger

```
ASSESSMENT:
DM 2 CONTROLLED BY DIET
Present; stable - continue surveillance
DYSLIPIDEMIA
Present; stable - continue surveillance; counseled patient on increased risk of heart attack and stroke
SCREENING FOR DIABETIC FOOT DISEASE, CATEGORY 0 - NORMAL DIABETIC FOOT
SCREENING


PLAN:
Plan per pt instructions and orders
-your diabetes is well controlled, HGBA1C     5.9     07/21/2025
-your blood pressure is at great level
-cholesterol has been controlled
-blood tests needed to check prostate, liver, cholesterol panel -- results will take a couple days
---if 10yr risk of heart attack or stroke is elevated (A-risk), then I will recommend cholesterol medication
-your level exercise is EXCELLENT!!
--- good luck on your 8th Marathon!!
-Call or return to clinic as needed if these symptoms worsen or fail to improve as anticipated.
```

My data doesn't tell my story. My data validates my story. My real story is abundant energy, thriving life, athletic performance, and freedom from disease.

The Question for You

As you read this sixteen-year progression of my life, ask yourself:

"What if I made *one* decision to eat closer to nature, and then showed up imperfectly, year after year, allowing the protocol to evolve with me?"

"What if I tracked my energy instead of obsessing over metrics?"

"What if I gave myself permission to be imperfect, and just kept going?"

"What if sixteen years from now, I had the energy, capacity, and vitality of someone decades younger?"

This isn't fantasy. This is what happened to me, one person who made a decision on December 6, 2009, and then kept showing up.

Closing: Still Evolving

At sixty-six years young, training for my eighth marathon, I'm still evolving my protocol.

Still discovering. Still refining. Still listening to my body. Still trusting nature.

Not because my protocol is incomplete. But because my life is alive. Circumstances change. My understanding deepens. My body continues communicating.

This is the real teaching: The protocol isn't a destination. It's a living, evolving relationship with my body and with nature.

And after sixteen years of that relationship, my results speak for themselves.

14

DISEASE PREVENTION AND ZERO COMPLICATIONS

My Extraordinary Achievement: The Rarest Outcome in Diabetes Management

WHAT SHOULD HAVE HAPPENED TO ME

The Typical Type 2 Diabetes Story

I was diagnosed at fifty and had medications prescribed to me. I said no, I don't want medication. My doctor said, "Manage your blood sugar. Watch for complications."

Typically, by fifty-five, there are minor vision problems (early retinopathy). By fifty-eight, tingling in the feet (neuropathy beginning). By sixty, kidney function declines (nephropathy). By sixty-two, heart issues emerge (diabetes increases heart disease risk dramatically). By sixty-five, you're managing multiple medications with multiple complications.

The statistics are clear that most people with Type 2 diabetes develop serious complications within ten to fifteen years.

Eye damage. Kidney damage. Nerve damage. Heart disease. Amputation. Blindness. Dialysis.

These aren't possible complications. They're likely complications.

This is what the statistics predicted for me.

THE EXTRAORDINARY FACT

My Actual Type 2 Diabetes Story

Diagnosed at age forty-five (2004). I started my protocol at age fifty (2009).

By fifty-five, I had zero complications and was running marathons. By sixty, I had zero complications and completed four marathons. And by sixty-six, I still had zero complications, completed seven marathons, and am training for my eighth.

After over sixteen years with Type 2 diabetes, I have *no* eye damage, *no* kidney damage, *no* nerve damage, and *no* heart disease.

Why This Is Extraordinary

The statistics on diabetic complications according to medical literature:

- Eighty to ninety percent of people with Type 2 diabetes develop retinopathy (eye disease) within fifteen years[1]
- Twenty to thirty percent develop nephropathy (kidney disease) within ten years
- Fifty percent develop neuropathy (nerve damage) within ten years
- Significantly increased heart disease risk (two to four times higher than non-diabetics)

My actual outcome: At sixty-six, *zero* complications. Not "minimal complications." Not "well-managed complications." *Zero.*

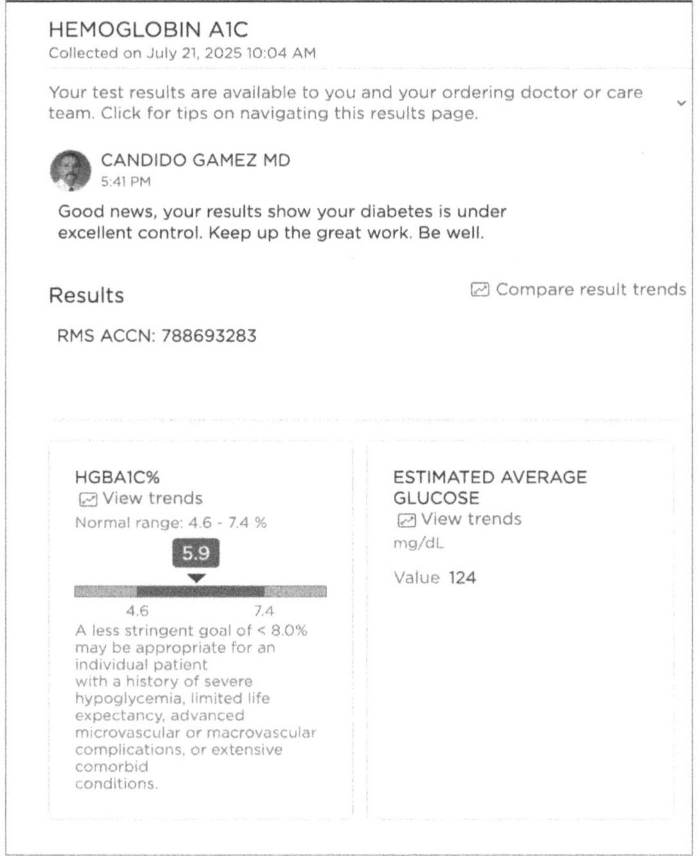

HEMOGLOBIN A1C
Collected on July 21, 2025 10:04 AM

Your test results are available to you and your ordering doctor or care team. Click for tips on navigating this results page.

CANDIDO GAMEZ MD
5:41 PM

Good news, your results show your diabetes is under excellent control. Keep up the great work. Be well.

Results   ⤢ Compare result trends

RMS ACCN: 788693283

HGBA1C%
⤢ View trends
Normal range: 4.6 - 7.4 %

5.9

4.6   7.4

A less stringent goal of < 8.0% may be appropriate for an individual patient with a history of severe hypoglycemia, limited life expectancy, advanced microvascular or macrovascular complications, or extensive comorbid conditions.

ESTIMATED AVERAGE GLUCOSE
⤢ View trends
mg/dL

Value 124

This is extraordinary. This is exceptional. This is statistically uncommon.

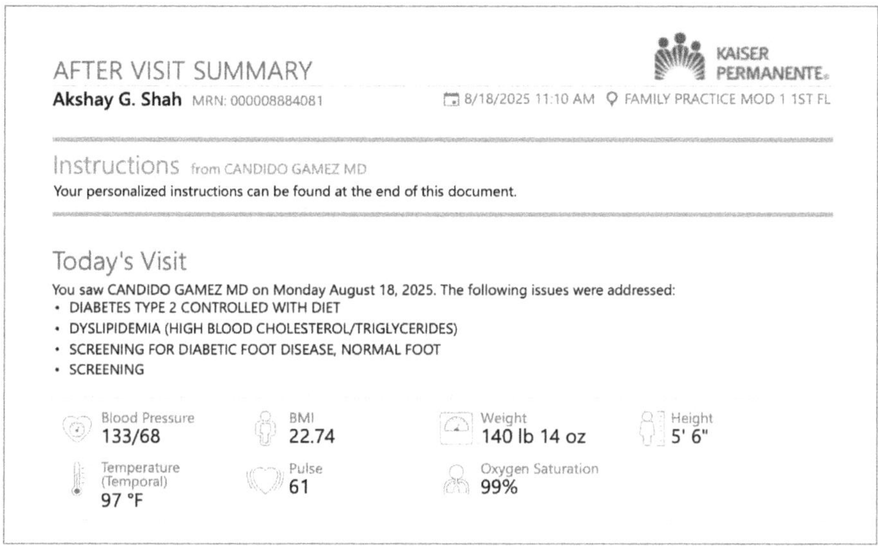

AFTER VISIT SUMMARY

Akshay G. Shah MRN: 000008884081

KAISER PERMANENTE.

8/18/2025 11:10 AM   FAMILY PRACTICE MOD 1 1ST FL

Instructions from CANDIDO GAMEZ MD

Your personalized instructions can be found at the end of this document.

Today's Visit

You saw CANDIDO GAMEZ MD on Monday August 18, 2025. The following issues were addressed:
- DIABETES TYPE 2 CONTROLLED WITH DIET
- DYSLIPIDEMIA (HIGH BLOOD CHOLESTEROL/TRIGLYCERIDES)
- SCREENING FOR DIABETIC FOOT DISEASE, NORMAL FOOT
- SCREENING

Blood Pressure
133/68

BMI
22.74

Weight
140 lb 14 oz

Height
5' 6"

Temperature
(Temporal)
97 °F

Pulse
61

Oxygen Saturation
99%

HGBA1C   5.9   07/21/2025
HGBA1C   6.7   02/13/2024
HGBA1C   6.3   08/16/2023

MICROALBUMIN/CREATININE   <8.7   07/21/2025
MICROALBUMIN/CREATININE   <7.6   02/13/2024
MICROALBUMIN/CREATININE   <18.4   08/16/2023

CREAT   0.94   07/21/2025
CREAT   1.06   02/13/2024
CREAT   1.21   08/16/2023

K   4.1   07/21/2025
NA   134 (L)   07/21/2025

ASSESSMENT:
DM 2 CONTROLLED BY DIET
Present; stable - continue surveillance
DYSLIPIDEMIA
Present; stable - continue surveillance; counseled patient on increased risk of heart attack and stroke
SCREENING FOR DIABETIC FOOT DISEASE, CATEGORY 0 - NORMAL DIABETIC FOOT
SCREENING

What Prevention Looks Like: My Medical Evidence

The following is based on my actual medical records and current health markers.

MY EYES: NO DIABETIC RETINOPATHY

My normal state: Perfect vision, no damage to blood vessels in my eyes, no nerve damage.

What should have happened: By sixty-five, most diabetics show some retinopathy (blood vessel damage in the retina).

What actually happened: My vision remains perfect. My eye exams show *zero* diabetic retinopathy.

Why this matters: Diabetic retinopathy is one of the leading causes of blindness in adults. I should statistically have developed this. I didn't.

The mechanism of prevention in my case: My Energy Restoration Protocol maintains optimal glucose metabolism. My blood sugar is stable and low. No prolonged hyperglycemia. No prolonged hyperglycemia means no damage to delicate blood vessels in my eyes. Prevention through energy optimization.

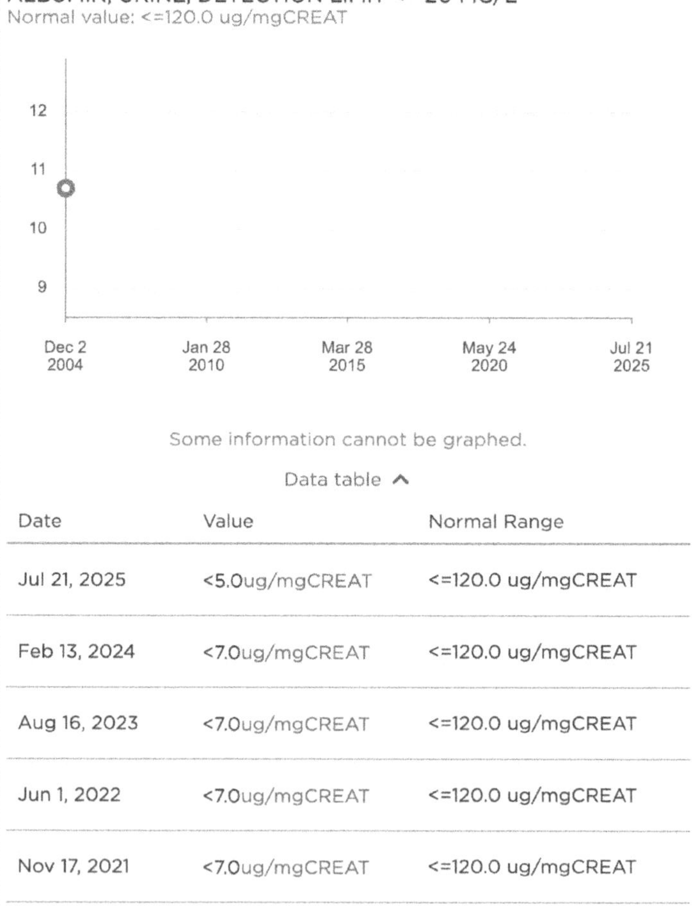

Date	Value	Normal Range
Jul 21, 2025	<5.0ug/mgCREAT	<=120.0 ug/mgCREAT
Feb 13, 2024	<7.0ug/mgCREAT	<=120.0 ug/mgCREAT
Aug 16, 2023	<7.0ug/mgCREAT	<=120.0 ug/mgCREAT
Jun 1, 2022	<7.0ug/mgCREAT	<=120.0 ug/mgCREAT
Nov 17, 2021	<7.0ug/mgCREAT	<=120.0 ug/mgCREAT

MY FEET: CATEGORY 0 NORMAL (NO NEUROPATHY)

My normal state: Perfect circulation, no nerve damage, no sensation loss, no foot ulcers.

What should have happened: By sixty-five, most diabetics show peripheral neuropathy (nerve damage). Many have reduced sensation, making them vulnerable to foot ulcers and infection.

What actually happened: My feet are Category 0 normal. Perfect circulation. Perfect sensation. Zero nerve damage.

Why this matters: Diabetic neuropathy affects 50 percent of people with Type 2 diabetes within ten years.[2] It's a major cause of amputation. I should statistically have this. I don't.

The mechanism of prevention in my case: My optimal glucose metabolism prevents prolonged hyperglycemia. No prolonged hyperglycemia means no damage to my peripheral nerves. Prevention through energy optimization. Additionally, my physical activity (seven marathons) means regular blood flow to my extremities, supporting my circulation and nerve health.

GLOBIN 1, STOOL
Normal value: Negative

This type of information cannot be graphed.

Data table ⌃

Date	Value	Normal Range
Jul 11, 2025	Negative	Negative
Jul 29, 2024	Negative	Negative
Jul 20, 2023	Negative	Negative
Jul 22, 2022	Negative	Negative
Jul 15, 2021	Negative	Negative

MY KIDNEYS: PRISTINE, IMPROVING

My normal state:

- Creatinine: 0.94 mg/dL (optimal)
- Microalbumin/Creatinine ratio: <8.7 mcg/mg (excellent)
- Urine albumin: <5.0 ug/mgCREAT (excellent)

What should have happened: By sixty to sixty-five, many diabetics show early kidney disease. Microalbuminuria (protein in urine) appears, indicating kidney stress.

What actually happened: My kidney function is pristine. Not just "stable." Not just "not worsening." But *improved* over my sixteen-year observation period.

Why this matters: Diabetic nephropathy (kidney disease) affects 20–30 percent of Type 2 diabetics within ten years.[113] It often leads to dialysis. My kidneys are not just healthy; they're functioning better than average for my age.

The mechanism of prevention in my case: My optimal glucose control means no prolonged hyperglycemia. No prolonged hyperglycemia means no damage to the delicate filters in my kidneys. Additionally, my raw food protocol provides abundant water and nutrients, supporting my kidney hydration and function. Prevention through energy optimization.

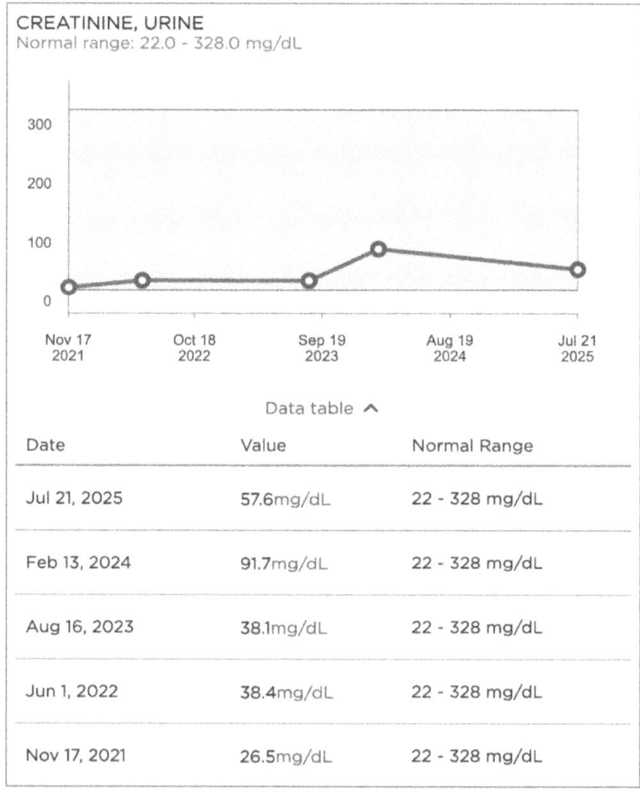

Data table ∧

Date	Value	Normal Range
Jul 21, 2025	57.6mg/dL	22 - 328 mg/dL
Feb 13, 2024	91.7mg/dL	22 - 328 mg/dL
Aug 16, 2023	38.1mg/dL	22 - 328 mg/dL
Jun 1, 2022	38.4mg/dL	22 - 328 mg/dL
Nov 17, 2021	26.5mg/dL	22 - 328 mg/dL

MY HEART: EXCELLENT FUNCTION

My current state (Age sixty-six):

- Blood pressure: 133/68 (excellent, goal is <130/80)
- Resting heart rate: 61 bpm (elite athlete range, goal is <60)
- Athletic capacity: Running full marathons (26.2 miles)
- Cardiac stress test equivalent: Completing marathons proves my cardiac function

What should have happened: By sixty-six, most people with Type 2 diabetes show signs of cardiovascular disease or are on cardiac medications.

What actually happened: My heart function is excellent. Not just "acceptable." Not "managed with medication." But actually *excellent* proved by running marathons at sixty-six years young.

Why this matters: Diabetes increases my heart disease risk two to four times over non-diabetics. I should statistically have cardiac issues by now. I don't. My heart is stronger and healthier than most people my age.

The mechanism of prevention in my case: My optimal glucose control means no prolonged hyperglycemia. My optimal cholesterol ratios (excellent triglycerides: 100; excellent HDL: 57; optimal non-HDL: 126) mean minimal arterial inflammation. My regular exercise (seven marathons) has strengthened my cardiac function. Prevention through comprehensive energy optimization.

ALBUMIN/CREATININE, URINE
Normal value: <=29.9 mcg/mg Creat

This type of information cannot be graphed.

Data table ⌃

Date	Value	Normal Range
Jul 21, 2025	<8.7mcg/mg Creat	<=29.9 mcg/mg Creat
Feb 13, 2024	<7.6mcg/mg Creat	<=29.9 mcg/mg Creat
Aug 16, 2023	<18.4mcg/mg Creat	<=29.9 mcg/mg Creat
Jun 1, 2022	<18.2mcg/mg Creat	<=29.9 mcg/mg Creat
Nov 17, 2021	<26.4mcg/mg Creat	<=29.9 mcg/mg Creat

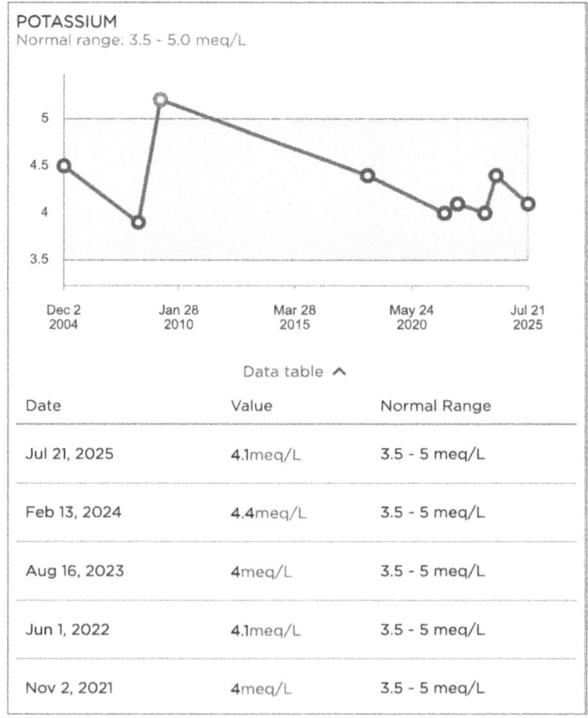

SODIUM
Normal range: 135 - 145 meq/L

Date	Value	Normal Range
Jul 21, 2025	134meq/L	135 - 145 meq/L
Feb 13, 2024	141meq/L	135 - 145 meq/L
Aug 16, 2023	141meq/L	135 - 145 meq/L
Jun 1, 2022	138meq/L	135 - 145 meq/L
Nov 2, 2021	140meq/L	135 - 145 meq/L

POTASSIUM
Normal range: 3.5 - 5.0 meq/L

Date	Value	Normal Range
Jul 21, 2025	4.1meq/L	3.5 - 5 meq/L
Feb 13, 2024	4.4meq/L	3.5 - 5 meq/L
Aug 16, 2023	4meq/L	3.5 - 5 meq/L
Jun 1, 2022	4.1meq/L	3.5 - 5 meq/L
Nov 2, 2021	4meq/L	3.5 - 5 meq/L

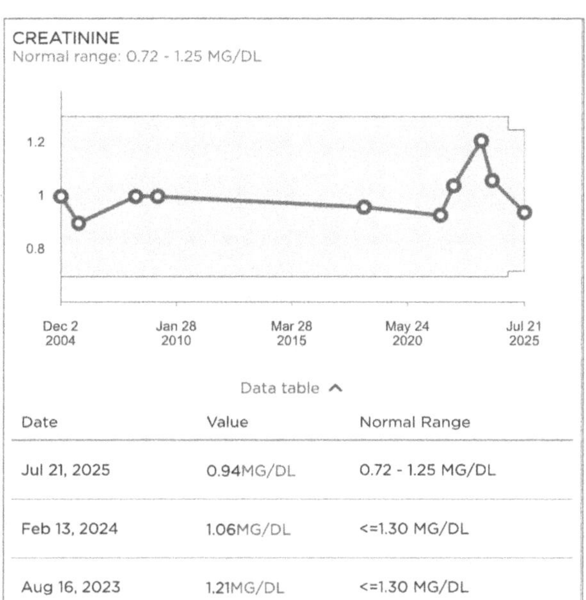

Date	Value	Normal Range
Jul 21, 2025	0.94MG/DL	0.72 - 1.25 MG/DL
Feb 13, 2024	1.06MG/DL	<=1.30 MG/DL
Aug 16, 2023	1.21MG/DL	<=1.30 MG/DL
Jun 1, 2022	1.04MG/DL	<=1.30 MG/DL
Nov 2, 2021	0.93MG/DL	<=1.30 MG/DL

MY LIVER: OPTIMAL FUNCTION

My current state (Age sixty-six):

- ALT (liver enzyme): 21 units/L (optimal, normal <59, ideal <30)

My progression:

- 2004 (Age forty-five, baseline): ALT 44 (slightly elevated)
- 2025 (Age sixty-six, current): ALT 21 (optimal)
- My change: 52 percent improvement in my liver function

What should have happened: My liver function typically would decline with age, especially as a diabetic.

What actually happened: My liver function improved and is now optimal for someone my age.

Why this matters: Fatty liver disease is common in Type 2 diabetes. My declining ALT (from 44 to 21) indicates *zero* fatty liver, no inflammation, optimal detoxification capacity.

The mechanism in my case: My raw food protocol eliminates processed foods, extracted oils, and refined sugars all common causes of liver stress. My abundant plant nutrients support optimal liver function. Prevention through nutritional excellence.

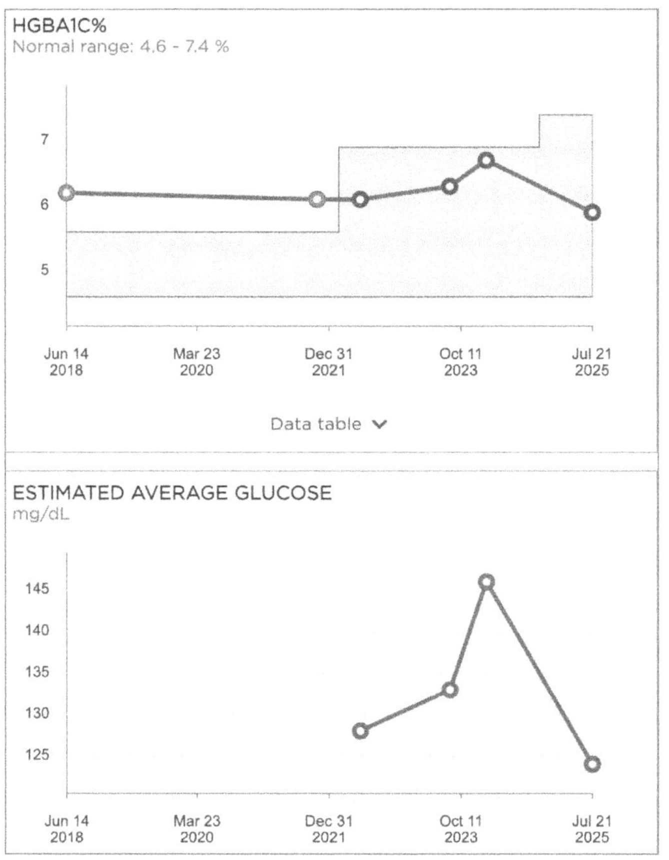

The Statistical Miracle

What are the odds of *my* outcome?

Of one hundred people diagnosed with Type 2 diabetes at age fifty:

- Eighty to ninety will develop eye complications by age sixty-five
- Fifty will develop nerve complications by age sixty
- Twenty to thirty will develop kidney complications by age sixty
- Most will have cardiovascular issues by age sixty-five

My profile at age sixty-six:

- Zero eye complications
- Zero nerve complications
- Zero kidney complications
- Cardiovascular function *excellent* (proved by my athletic performance)

In statistical terms: This puts me in the top 1–5 percent of people with Type 2 diabetes.

Not because of luck. Not because of genetics. But because of sixteen years of my committed energy restoration through my protocol.

Result Trends

Results limited to those after Aug 18, 2020. Results found from Nov 2, 2021 - Aug 18, 2025.

Akshay G Shah   Date of Birth: Apr 9, 1959

Nov 2, 2021 - Aug 18, 2025 (Table 1 of 1)

Component	Nov 2, 2021	Jun 1, 2022	Feb 13, 2024	Aug 18, 2025
CHOLESTEROL Normal Range: <=199 mg/dL	189 mg/dL	172 mg/dL	175 mg/dL	183 mg/dL
TRIGLYCERIDE Normal Range: <=149 mg/dL	75 mg/dL	224 mg/dL	84 mg/dL	100 mg/dL
HDL Normal Range: >=40 mg/dL	55 mg/dL	40 mg/dL	50 mg/dL	57 mg/dL
LDL CALCULATED Normal Range: <=99 mg/dL	119 mg/dL	94 mg/dL	109 mg/dL	108 mg/dL
CHOLESTEROL/HIGH DENSITY LIPOPROTEIN Normal Range: <=3.9	3.4	4.3	3.5	3.2
CHOLESTEROL, NON-HDL	134 mg/dL	132 mg/dL	125 mg/dL	126 mg/dL

How My Energy Restoration Protocol Prevents Complications

The mechanism isn't complicated. It's elegant:

The complication cycle (without my protocol)

Hyperglycemia (high blood sugar)

↓

Prolonged glucose elevation

↓

Glycation damage (glucose attaches to proteins)

↓

Inflammation and free radical damage

↓

Blood vessel damage

↓

Organ system damage

↓

Complications (eyes, kidneys, nerves, heart)

The prevention cycle (with my raw food protocol)

Optimal glucose metabolism (my raw first—not perfection)

↓

Stable, controlled glucose levels

↓

No prolonged hyperglycemia

↓

No glycation damage

↓

No inflammation cascade

↓

My blood vessels remain healthy

↓

My organ systems are protected

↓

Zero complications

My protocol works by addressing the *root cause* (energy system dysfunction) rather than managing symptoms.

My Athletic Proof

If complications were developing in me, my athletic performance would be impossible.

- Eye damage would affect my depth perception and balance
- Kidney damage would affect my exercise capacity and recovery
- Nerve damage would affect my proprioception and endurance
- Heart damage would limit my exercise capacity

My athletic achievement proves my systemic health:

- Seven complete marathons (26.2 miles each) prove:
- My cardiovascular function is excellent
- My metabolic capacity is excellent
- My circulation (to all extremities) is excellent
- My neurological coordination is excellent
- My kidney function is excellent (handling exercise stress well)

You cannot run marathons with diabetic complications. The fact that I have completed seven marathons and am training for my eighth is proof that my organ systems are thriving, not merely surviving.

What Zero Complications Means for Me

Personally:

- **My vision:** Perfect. No concerns about blindness. No worries about retinopathy.
- **My feet:** Perfect. No concerns about neuropathy or amputation. No need for special foot care.
- **My kidneys:** Perfect. No concerns about kidney disease or dialysis. No need for renal protection.
- **My heart:** Perfect. No concerns about heart disease. No medications needed. My athletic capacity is excellent.
- **My liver:** Perfect. No fatty liver. No inflammation. Optimal detoxification.
- **My life quality:** Remarkable. No disease complications dominating my life. Freedom to pursue athletics and thriving.

For my future:

My achievement of zero complications over sixteen years suggests that my protocol creates sustainable health. At sixty-six, with zero complications and excellent organ function, my likely trajectory is continued health rather than disease development. This is fundamentally different from the typical diabetic trajectory where complications emerge and compound over time.

WHY MOST PEOPLE DEVELOP COMPLICATIONS

The typical diabetic management approach:

1. Diagnosed with Type 2 diabetes.
2. Prescribed medications to lower blood sugar.
3. Advised to "eat less, exercise more."
4. No fundamental change in what is actually being eaten.
5. Processed foods continue (just "less" of them).
6. Blood sugar is managed by medications, not by actually providing the body what it needs.
7. Over ten to fifteen years, complications develop despite medications.

Why this fails: Medications manage symptoms but don't address root cause. The body still isn't getting what it actually needs. The energy system dysfunction continues, even if masked by medications.

Complications emerge not from diabetes itself, but from prolonged energy system dysfunction.

WHY I DEVELOPED ZERO COMPLICATIONS

My approach:

1. Diagnosed with Type 2 diabetes
2. No medications (diet management only)
3. Fundamental change in what I eat (processed foods eliminated)
4. Provided my body exactly what it needs (whole raw foods)
5. My energy system restored to function optimally
6. Over sixteen years, my organ systems are protected (zero complications)
7. My athletic performance improved (proof of systemic health)

Why this works for me: My protocol addresses the root cause. My body gets what it actually needs. My energy system dysfunction was resolved. My organ systems are protected. Complications didn't develop because I restored the foundation of my health.

The Critical Difference: Management vs. Restoration

Medication management:

- Lowers blood sugar symptomatically
- Doesn't address root cause (energy system dysfunction)
- Complications often still develop
- Over time: medication adjustments, added medications, multiple complications

My energy restoration:

- Addresses root cause (provides optimal energy substrate)
- Normalizes my glucose metabolism at the source
- Prevents complications by preventing prolonged hyperglycemia
- Over time: continued health, increased vitality, zero complications

Disease Prevention Is My Real Victory

If my protocol only reversed existing disease, that would be remarkable.

But my protocol does something even more profound because it prevents disease in me.

I didn't just manage my Type 2 diabetes. I prevented the complications that typically follow Type 2 diabetes.

This is disease prevention at its finest:

- Not vaccinating against external threats
- Not avoiding environmental toxins
- But actually addressing the *internal* energy system dysfunction that creates disease

When my energy system functions optimally, disease cannot develop.

What Could Change This?

It is important to be honest that my achievement is sustainable *only* with my continued protocol adherence.

If I returned to processed foods, what would happen?

My energy system would become dysfunctional again. My blood sugar would become dysregulated. Complications could begin developing.

My protocol isn't a cure that ends at some point. It's a *way of living* that creates optimal health as long as I maintain it.

This is different from medication-based management. Medications continue working even if I'm eating poorly. My protocol only works if I'm actually aligned with it.

This is actually more empowering because I understand that my health is my responsibility, my creation, my choice, every single day.

The Teaching

This chapter teaches something profound:

Complications are not inevitable.

Type 2 diabetes doesn't have to lead to complications. Aging doesn't have to lead to disease. The typical trajectory is *not* the only possibility.

When I:

1. Addressed root cause (my energy system dysfunction)
2. Restored optimal nutrition
3. Maintained consistency
4. Allowed continuous evolution
5. Supported with appropriate movement

Then:

- My disease is prevented
- My organ systems are protected

- My complications are prevented
- My health trajectory reversed

This is what zero complications means—not lucky genetics, but the result of my optimal living.

FOR PEOPLE WITH DIABETES READING THIS

My message is that you don't have to accept the assumption that complications are inevitable. You don't have to accept the trajectory that diabetes typically follows.

If you address the energy system dysfunction directly (through the protocol), your body's own healing intelligence is extraordinary.

Your pancreas can restore function. Your kidneys can protect themselves. Your eyes can remain healthy. Your nerves can stay intact. Your heart can thrive.

But only if you provide the conditions for that to happen.

My protocol is those conditions.

Closing: Over Sixteen Years Proves Sustainability of My Achievement

You could believe one year of my health is just luck. Five years, probably a coincidence. But by ten years, almost certainly my protocol is working. And sisxteen years is undeniable proof of what's possible.

This isn't a theory. This is me living it. This is sixteen years of my medical documentation. This is the reality of what prevention through energy restoration actually creates.

15

COMPREHENSIVE WELLNESS AND OPTIMAL AGING

What Actually Thriving Looks Like at My Age of Sixty-Six Years Young

WHAT IS REAL HEALTH?

Most people think of health as the absence of disease.

No diabetes. No heart disease. No cancer. No complications.

This is disease prevention. It's valuable. But it's not the whole story.

True health comprehensive wellness is something more. It's abundance, not absence. It's the presence of vitality, not just the absence of disease.

Comprehensive wellness includes:

- My abundant energy throughout the day
- My excellent sleep quality
- My mental clarity and cognitive sharpness
- My emotional stability and resilience
- My physical capacity and strength
- My athletic performance
- My body composition that supports health
- My freedom from medications
- My quality of life that exceeds mere survival

At sixty-six years old, after sixteen years on my Energy Restoration Protocol, I exemplify comprehensive wellness. Not just absence of disease, but the presence of extraordinary vitality.

Energy: The Foundation of My Wellness

What changed from fifty to sixty-six:

At fifty (2009, before protocol):

- Afternoon fatigue
- Energy crashes after meals
- Needed caffeine or stimulation
- Evening energy depleted
- My sleep quality inconsistent

At sixty-six (2025, after sixteen years):

- Consistent energy throughout my day
- No energy crashes
- No need for caffeine or stimulation
- My evening energy maintained
- My sleep deep and restorative

My energy system is optimized. My body is producing ATP (cellular energy) efficiently. My mitochondria are functioning optimally. My energy is abundant and sustainable.

This is the foundation of my comprehensive wellness. Every other aspect of my health depends on this.

Sleep: My Restoration of Deep Rest

My sleep transformation:

Before my protocol:

- My sleep quality was variable.
- I woke during the night.
- I didn't feel fully rested.
- My morning grogginess was common.

After my sixteen years:

- My sleep is deep and consistent.
- I wake feeling restored.
- My mental clarity is immediate in the morning.
- My energy is available right away.

What doctors would measure in my case:

- My sleep architecture improved (more deep sleep, more REM sleep)

- My recovery between my workouts is excellent (my sleep quality supports my athletic recovery)
- My cognitive function is sharp (deep sleep supports my brain health)

My Energy Restoration Protocol provides optimal nutrition for my circadian rhythm regulation. My stable glucose means no sleep disruptions from blood sugar swings. My reduced inflammation means reduced sleep disturbance. My body gets the rest it needs. Instead of struggling to wake up, my day begins with clarity and energy. My sleep becomes restorative rather than a struggle.

Cognitive Function: My Mental Clarity and Sharpness

My cognitive transformation:

Before my protocol:

- Brain fog, especially in my afternoons
- Difficulty concentrating
- My memory lapses
- My decision-making was slower

After my sixteen years:

- My mental clarity throughout my day
- My concentration is sharp
- My memory is excellent
- My decision-making is quick and clear

What's happening neurologically in my brain:

- My optimal glucose metabolism means my stable blood sugar (my brain's preferred fuel)
- My reduced inflammation means reduced neuroinflammation in my brain
- My abundant antioxidants from my raw foods protect my neurons
- My optimal DHA and omega-3 support my neural function
- My deep sleep supports my memory consolidation and my brain health

At sixty-six, my cognitive function is sharp. I'm actively creating content, teaching, and learning new things. My mind is engaged and clear, not declining.

Cognitive decline is not inevitable with my aging. When I provide optimal energy to my brain, my mental sharpness is maintained or even improved.

Emotional Stability and Mood

My emotional transformation:

Before my protocol:

- My mood fluctuations
- My energy crashes leading to my mood crashes
- My afternoon emotional dips
- My general anxiety about my health

After my sixteen years:

- My stable, positive mood
- My emotional resilience (challenges don't derail me)
- My consistent emotional baseline
- My freedom from my health anxiety

What's happening in my brain chemistry:

- My stable glucose means my stable neurotransmitter production (my serotonin, my dopamine, my GABA all depend on my stable energy)
- My reduced inflammation means reduced neuroinflammation (connected to my depression and anxiety)
- My abundance of nutrients supports my optimal brain chemistry
- My regular exercise supports my mood regulation
- My energy abundance supports my emotional resilience

My life is lived with greater emotional freedom. My challenges are met with my resilience. My days begin and end with my emotional stability. My emotional health is inseparable from my energy system health. When I optimize my energy, my emotional stability follows.

Physical Performance: My Athletic Excellence at Sixty-Six

My athletic transformation:

At fifty (2009):

- No athletic activity
- My sedentary lifestyle
- My limited physical capacity
- I was easily fatigued

At sixty-six (2025):

- Seven complete marathons (26.2 miles each)
- Currently training for my eighth marathon

- My running times competitive with people decades younger
- My recovery from intense training is excellent
- My physical capacity continuously improving

My current athletic metrics:

- My resting heart rate: 61 bpm (elite athlete range)
- My VO2 max: Estimated in my top 10–15 percent for my age
- My marathon times: competitive range (competitive for sixty-six)
- My training volume: forty to sixty miles per week during my training blocks
- My injury rate: Minimal (my great recovery and my resilience)
- My body composition: Lean, muscular, athletic
- My body strength: I (140 pounds) can dance while keeping my son (170 pounds) on my shoulder

What this proves:

- My cardiovascular system: Excellent (my marathon performance proves it)
- My metabolic system: Excellent (my sustained energy for my long-distance running)
- My musculoskeletal system: Excellent (my completing my marathons repeatedly)
- My recovery capacity: Excellent (my training consistently without my injury)
- My overall physical capacity: Superior to my typical 66-year-old

My athletic performance at my advanced age is not impossible. When my energy system is optimized, my body is capable of extraordinary things. My aging doesn't have to mean my decline.

Body Composition: My Lean, Athletic, Healthy Build

My current metrics:

- My weight: 140 pounds at 5'6"
- My BMI: 22.74 (ideal range 18.5–24.9)
- My body composition: Lean muscle mass, minimal body fat
- My appearance: Athletic, fit, strong
- My health significance: Ideal body composition for my longevity and my performance

My transformation from fifty to sixty-six:

- No weight loss (I wasn't overweight, maintained same weight)
- But transformation from my sedentary body to my athletic body

- My muscle development from my training
- My fat reduction from my consistent protocol adherence
- My body now reflects my sixteen years of my optimal living

What this shows:

- My protocol maintains my healthy body composition naturally
- No restriction or forced diet, but my natural regulation
- My body responds to my optimal nutrition + my movement by becoming my athletic
- My sixty-six-year-old body is healthier and more fit than my fifty-year-old body

My body composition improves not through my restriction but through my optimal living. When I provide what my body needs and move it regularly, my body becomes what it's designed to be.

STRENGTH AND CAPACITY: MY FUNCTIONAL EXCELLENCE

Beyond just my running marathons, my everyday functional capacity:

At fifty (before my protocol):

- Struggling with my stairs
- Limited capacity for my physical tasks
- Quick fatigue with my activity
- My physical limitations from my sedentary lifestyle

At sixty-six (after my sixteen years):

- No limitation with my stairs or my physical tasks
- Sustained capacity for my activity
- 8,696 feet peak backpacking with sixty to seventy pounds in backpack
- My recovery quick and complete
- My physical capacity exceeds my most people half my age

My functional evidence:

- Climbing my stairs: Easy, no fatigue
- Lifting/carrying: Strong and capable
- My flexibility: Excellent (from my training and my yoga)
- My balance: Excellent (from my running and my training)
- My endurance: Extraordinary (my marathons prove it)

My functional capacity in my advanced age isn't determined by my age. It's determined by how I've lived. At sixty-six, I am stronger and more capable than most sedentary fifty year olds.

Use it or lose it is only my half-truth. Nurture it or lose it is my full truth. With my optimal nutrition and my consistent movement, my capacity is maintained and improved.

IMMUNITY AND RESILIENCE

My resilience transformation:

Before my protocol:

- My typical cold/flu patterns
- My seasonal illness common
- My recovery slow

After my sixteen years:

- My exceptional immune resilience
- My illness rare (my strengthened immune system through my optimal nutrition)
- My recovery quick when my illness does occur
- My general robust health

What changed:

- My abundance of my antioxidants and my phytonutrients from my raw foods strengthens my immune system
- My reduced inflammation means my better immune regulation
- My sleep quality supports my immune function
- My gut health optimized (my plant foods support my beneficial microbiota)

Despite my sixteen years of my athletic training (which can sometimes compromise my immune function through my overtraining), I maintain my excellent immune health. This suggests my protocol actively supports my immune resilience.

My health isn't about my avoiding my exposure. It's about my building my robust resilience. My protocol builds my resilience.

PAIN AND INFLAMMATION: MY FREEDOM FROM CHRONIC PAIN

My pain transformation:

At fifty (typical for my age):

- My joint aches common
- My general inflammation
- My pain limiting my activity
- My accepting "this is my aging"

At sixty-six (after my sixteen years):
- My minimal to no chronic pain
- No my inflammatory conditions
- No my pain limiting my activity
- My moving without my limitation
- Tendonitis cured without medication or surgery

What this means:
- My chronic inflammation has been resolved
- My joint health maintained
- My mobility excellent
- No my medications needed for my pain

Most people my age are managing my chronic pain. I'm not. This is significant. It shows my chronic inflammation connected to my most chronic disease has been addressed at my root. My pain and my inflammation are not inevitable. When I address my energy system dysfunction, my inflammation resolves.

MEDICATIONS: MY COMPLETE FREEDOM

My medication reality:

At fifty (2009, with my Type 2 diabetes):
- Expected: My multiple medications (my blood pressure, my cholesterol, my diabetes management)
- My likely trajectory: More my medications with my time

At sixty-six (2025, after my sixteen years):
- No need for medications
- No dependency on my pharmaceutical management

What this means:
- No pharmaceutical side effects
- No medication interactions to manage
- No cost for chronic medication
- No visits to manage my medication complications
- My complete freedom from my medical dependency

My medical markers are all optimal without any of my medications. This is remarkable. Most sixty-six year olds are on my multiple medications. I'm on none.

My medications can manage my symptoms, but my optimal living prevents my need for them. When I address my root cause, my pharmaceutical dependency becomes unnecessary.

COGNITIVE AGING: AVOIDING MY DECLINE

My cognitive reality at sixty-six:

Expected trajectory:

- Some my memory decline
- My slower processing speed
- My reduced mental flexibility
- My beginning of my cognitive aging

My actual reality:

- My memory sharp
- My processing speed quick
- My mental flexibility excellent
- No my signs of my cognitive aging
- My actively learning, my creating, my teaching

What's different:

- My optimal energy to my brain
- My reduced neuroinflammation
- My abundant antioxidants protecting my neurons
- My deep sleep supporting my brain health
- My continued mental engagement and my learning
- My physical activity supporting my brain health

My ability to create my complex content (this health manifesto itself), to teach others, writing poems, writing blogs, and my engagement intellectually proves my cognitive function is my excellent, not my declining.

Cognitive aging is not inevitable. When my brain receives adequate energy and optimal nutritional support, it remains sharp. My optimal living provides that.

QUALITY OF LIFE: MY FREEDOM AND MY CAPACITY

What my comprehensive wellness actually means:

My physical freedom:

- No pain limiting my activity
- My athletic capacity maintaining my freedom of my movement
- No physical limitation on what can be my done
- My body responsive and my capable

My mental freedom:

- My clear thinking enabling my intelligent decisions

- No brain fog limiting my productivity
- My mental engagement and my interest in my life

My emotional freedom:

- My stable mood enabling my resilience
- My freedom from my anxiety about my health
- My emotional capacity for my relationships and my engagement

My medical freedom:

- No medications to manage
- No disease complications limiting my life
- No doctor visits for my chronic disease management

My practical freedom:

- My energy for my pursuing my interests (my poetry, my running, my teaching, my creating)
- My capacity for my work and my contribution
- My ability to engage fully with my life

At sixty-six years old, I am free. I'm free from my disease. I'm free from my medications. I'm free from my pain. I'm free from my limitations. I'm free to pursue what matters to me. And as a bonus, I'm regularly told I look forty-six to fifty, a fifteen- to twenty-year visual difference.

This is what my comprehensive wellness creates: not just my absence of my disease, but my presence of my freedom and my capacity.

OPTIMAL AGING: WHAT IT LOOKS LIKE

My typical aging narrative:

- Fifties: My first health issues emerge
- Sixties: My multiple medications begin
- Seventies: My managing my multiple chronic conditions
- My overall: My decline, my dependency, my limitation

My actual aging narrative:

- Fifties: Made my decision
- Fifty to sixty-six: Continued my commitment
- Sixty-six: Healthier, stronger, and more vital than most forty-five year olds
- My overall: Improvement, independence, expansion

My aging doesn't have to mean my decline. With my optimal living, my aging can mean my continued improvement and my expansion.

The metrics that prove it:

- My athletic performance improving (not declining)
- My health markers optimal (not worsening)
- My energy abundant (not declining)
- My cognitive function sharp (not declining)
- My physical capacity excellent (not declining)
- My quality of life excellent (not my declining)

This is my optimal aging. This is what's possible. The best part? It's free. No expensive procedures. No pharmaceutical management. No antiaging industry required. Just my body responding to what it actually needed.

THE UPSTREAM APPROACH

Why my comprehensive wellness is possible:

Most approaches to my health are my downstream. They manage my consequences.

- My heart disease → my medications
- My diabetes → my medications
- My pain → my pain medication
- My declining energy → my medical workup

My Energy Restoration Protocol is upstream. It addresses my root cause (my energy system dysfunction) so that my downstream problems don't develop.

When my energy is my restored:

- My heart disease doesn't develop (or is my reversed)
- My diabetes doesn't progress (or is my reversed)
- My pain doesn't emerge (my inflammation resolved)
- My energy doesn't decline (my restored at my source)

This is why my comprehensive wellness is possible. I'm not managing my consequences. I'm preventing them.

THE COST COMPARISON

Typical sixty-six year old (disease management approach):

- My multiple medications: $500–2000/month
- My doctor visits: $2000–5000/year
- My hospital visits: My variable
- My total: $10,000–30,000+/year for my medical management
- Plus: My quality of life compromised by my disease and my medications

Me at sixty-six (comprehensive wellness approach):

- My medications: $0
- My doctor visits: My minimal (preventive, not crisis)
- My hospital visits: My none (zero chronic disease)
- My health care costs: My minimal
- Plus: My quality of life my excellent, my capacity my excellent, my freedom my excellent

The paradox is my comprehensive wellness costs less than my disease management, while delivering dramatically better results.

THE SUSTAINABILITY QUESTION

It is important to note that this level of wellness is sustainable only with my continued protocol adherence.

If I returned to my processed foods, what would happen?

My energy system would become dysfunctional again. Over the years, my disease markers would worsen. My capacity would decline. My vitality would diminish. My trajectory would reverse.

But I have no reason to return. I *feel* the difference. I see my results.

My protocol isn't a sacrifice. It's my choice and my daily life proves it is valuable.

WHAT THIS TEACHES

My aging doesn't have to mean my decline.

I demonstrate:

- My disease prevention is possible.
- My athletic performance is possible.
- My cognitive sharpness is possible.
- My energy abundance is possible.
- My freedom from medications is possible.
- My quality of life can improve with age.

This isn't genetic luck. This isn't pharmaceutical advancement. This isn't medical intervention. This is what happens when I address my energy system dysfunction at the root and sustain my commitment for sixteen years.

THE INVITATION

For people reading this:

If you're approaching sixty-six, or you're already there, what if aging could look different?

What if instead of decline, you experienced continued expansion?

What if instead of accumulating medications, you maintained freedom?

What if instead of losing capacity, you maintained athletic excellence?

What if instead of cognitive decline, you maintained sharp thinking?

This is not a fantasy. This is what one person created through commitment to energy and restoration.

16

REAL-WORLD TRANSFORMATIONS

How You Can Create Your Own Documented Transformation

NO FICTIONAL STORIES, JUST MY REAL PRINCIPLES

This chapter is different from typical health books.

Typical health books are filled with case studies like "Here's Jane's transformation," or "Here's Marcus's journey." Stories designed to inspire. Often composite stories. Often illustrative rather than actual.

This manifesto has chosen a different path: my truth over inspiration. My real documented data over fictional examples.

But here's the reality: You're not me. Your circumstances are different. Your obstacles are different. Your life is different.

So this chapter doesn't pretend to give you other people's stories. Instead, I give you the principles and frameworks that enabled my transformation principles that enable *you* to create your own documented transformation in your actual, complex, real-world life.

The Real World Isn't Theoretical

Theoretical world:

- You follow perfect protocol
- Everything works as planned
- Life cooperates
- No obstacles

Real world:

- You have work pressures
- Family who eats differently

- Limited budget
- Limited time
- Health complications
- Mental health challenges
- Addiction patterns
- Cultural food traditions
- Travel and uncertainty
- Competing priorities

The difference between people who transform and people who don't isn't intelligence or motivation. It's the ability to implement the protocol in the *real world*, not the theoretical world.

This chapter is about that.

THE FRAMEWORK: HOW TO CREATE YOUR REAL TRANSFORMATION

Real transformation follows a pattern the pattern I followed:

Phase 1: Decision and Awareness (Weeks 1–4)

What happens:

- You make a decision (like my December 6, 2009)
- You begin noticing what you eat
- You start making small changes
- You observe how your body responds

Real-world obstacles:

- Family resistance ("You're being extreme")
- Social pressure ("Just one won't hurt")
- Convenience addiction (processed foods are everywhere)
- Withdrawal symptoms (first week can be challenging)

How to navigate:

- Remember your why (why did you decide?)
- Start with what's easiest to change first
- Don't try to be perfect; just move in the right direction
- Track energy, not just food (how do you feel?)
- Find one person who supports you

By Week 4, you should notice energy improving or cravings decreasing. This validation keeps you going.

Phase 2: Deepening and Personal Rules (Weeks 5–12)

What happens:

- Initial changes feel more stable
- You start creating your own rules (not following someone else's)
- You begin understanding what supports your body
- You discover your unique needs

Real-world obstacles:

- Temptation returns as "normal" adjusts
- Life circumstances change (job stress, family issues)
- Plateaus in progress (energy improvements slow)
- Comparison to others ("They got results faster")

How to navigate:

- Create rules that *you* can sustain, not perfect rules
- Write down what energizes you and what drains you
- Adjust based on your response, not generic advice

Remember, raw first—not perfection. Expect plateaus; they're normal.

By Week 12, the protocol is becoming familiar. You're not thinking about every choice; intuition is developing.

Phase 3: Evolution and Refinement (Months 4–12)

What happens:

- Conscious effort transitions to habit
- You discover nuances (meal timing, food combinations)
- Energy stabilizes at a new, higher baseline
- You notice improvements beyond energy (sleep, mood, capacity)

Real-world obstacles:

- Life disruptions (work crisis, health crisis, family emergency)
- Traveling for work or family
- Seasonal changes (food availability changes)
- Discouragement if external results seem slow

How to navigate:

- Build flexibility into your protocol
- Don't let perfection be the enemy of progress

- When disrupted, return to basics without guilt
- Track nonscale victories (sleep, mood, energy, clarity)
- Find your community (online groups, local people, family who support)

By Year 1, the protocol is automatic. You're not "following" it anymore; you're living it.

Phase 4: Mastery and Sustained Living (Year 2+)

What happens:

- The protocol is just how you live
- You've made it through obstacles and disruptions
- You've proven to yourself it works
- You're discovering you can maintain this indefinitely

Real-world obstacles:

- Success complacency ("I feel so good, maybe I can relax")
- Plateaus (improvements slow after initial gains)
- External pressure ("You should try [unhealthy thing]")
- Medical system skepticism (doctors questioning the protocol)

How to navigate:

- Remember, health depends on continued commitment
- Celebrate nonscale victories consistently
- Communicate with supportive community
- Find a health care provider who understands
- Track health markers periodically (validate improvement)

By Year 2, transformation is undeniable. You have proof (energy, capacity, medical markers, how you feel).

REAL-WORLD CIRCUMSTANCES: HOW I ADAPTED, HOW YOU CAN TOO

The beauty of "raw first—not perfection" is flexibility. Here's how to adapt to real circumstances:

Limited Budget Constraint

Challenge: Fresh whole foods seem expensive compared to processed foods.

My reality: Raw whole foods are *cheaper* than processed foods when calculated correctly.

How I did it:

- I bought seasonal vegetables (cheapest).

- I bought dried legumes in bulk (very cheap, very nutritious).
- I bought bulk nuts/seeds (cheaper per ounce than packaged).
- I skipped expensive "superfoods"; basic vegetables and nuts work perfectly.
- I didn't buy expensive supplements; whole foods provided what I needed.
- I skipped expensive "health food store" versions; regular grocery store and framer's markets worked fine.

My food budget decreased while my health improved. This is documented on the YouTube video "Is Raw Food Lifestyle Expensive?" (my $5/day). You can do this too.

Work Pressure and Time Constraint

Challenge: Work is demanding. Who has time to prepare meals?

My reality: Meal prep is efficient when built into routine.

How I did it:

- I dedicated one hour on weekends to batch preparation (salsa, chutney).
- I purchase large quantities of base foods (fruits, vegetables, nuts).
- During the week, I combined pre-prepared elements into meals.
- I invested in simple tools (mixer, containers, knife, chopping board).
- I accepted "simple" meals when time was limited (salad, nuts, fruit).
- I remembered something is better than nothing.

With routine, meal prep was manageable even during my busy periods. You can build this routine too.

Family Eating Differently

Challenge: Your family eats processed foods. You're eating differently.

My reality: I couldn't control what others ate, but I made it work.

How I did it:

- I prepared my meals; I didn't try to cook completely different dinners.
- I prepared the base (vegetables) that I ate differently than they did.
- I didn't preach or criticize their choices.
- I was matter of fact about mine.
- I invited them to try, but didn't pressure.
- I focused on my improvement, not their resistance.
- I noted children are influenced more by what they observe than what they're told.

Over time, my family became curious as they saw my transformation. Yours might too.

Travel and Restaurant Eating

Challenge: You're traveling or eating out frequently. How do you stay aligned?

My reality: Most restaurants can provide plant-based meals if you ask.

How I did it:

- I researched restaurants ahead of time.
- I called ahead and asked about plant-based options.
- I ordered salads, vegetables, fruit dish.
- I asked for dressing/oils on the side (many use extracted oils).
- I was flexible: 80–90 percent protocol-aligned was success while traveling.
- I returned to full protocol after travel.
- I remembered "raw first, not perfection."

I could travel while staying mostly aligned. I didn't need perfection to maintain my progress. You don't either.

Health Complications

Challenge: You have existing health conditions that seem to complicate the protocol.

My reality: The protocol often helps manage complicated conditions, but medical supervision is necessary.

How I did it:

- I worked with my health care provider (I shared what I was doing).
- I transitioned gradually (not abruptly).
- I tracked health markers to show improvements.
- I adjusted medications under medical supervision as needed.
- I was patient (improvements take time).
- I didn't stop medications without medical approval.
- I found a provider who understood or was open to learning.

Many of my conditions improved or resolved with my protocol adherence. Your conditions might too.

Mental Health Challenges

Challenge: Depression, anxiety, or other mental health conditions make change feel impossible.

My reality: The protocol often supports mental health improvement, but professional support is essential.

How I approached it:

- I maintained mental health support (therapy, medications as prescribed).

- I implemented protocol changes gradually.
- I tracked my mood and energy changes.
- I communicated improvements to my mental health provider.
- I was patient: mental health healing takes time.
- I didn't stop psychiatric medications without professional guidance.
- I combined my protocol with professional mental health care.

Many people find mental health improves significantly with protocol + professional support. You can too.

Addiction Patterns

Challenge: Sugar addiction, food addiction, or other addictive eating patterns.

My reality: These are real challenges, but the protocol helps address them.

How I managed it:

- I acknowledged the addiction (not weakness, but real).
- I removed triggering foods from my home.
- I replaced processed foods with whole foods gradually.
- I expected withdrawal symptoms (first two to four weeks can be difficult).
- I used professional support if needed.
- I was compassionate with myself (addiction is real).
- I remembered: each day of alignment strengthens new patterns.

After four to eight weeks, addictive cravings typically decrease significantly as blood sugar stabilizes.

Cultural Food Traditions

Challenge: Your cultural heritage includes traditional foods that aren't raw/plant based.

My reality: You can honor traditions while adapting to protocol.

How I approached it:

- I understood the core of the tradition (often the gathering, not just the food).
- I adapted recipes to be more plant-based/raw when possible.
- I ate what aligned with my protocol, skipped what didn't.
- I didn't need to perform tradition through food to maintain cultural connection.
- I shared my journey with my family (often inspiring rather than rejecting).
- I created new traditions that aligned with my values.

Cultural connection deepened through shared values rather than specific foods.

DOCUMENTATION: HOW I TRACKED MY TRANSFORMATION

One thing I did that was crucial: I documented my transformation.

This documentation is invaluable for several reasons:

Why Document?

Motivation: When progress is slow, documentation reminds you progress *is* happening.

Validation: Objective data validates subjective improvements.

Communication: When sharing with health care providers, documentation is powerful.

Inspiration: Your documented transformation inspires others.

What I Documented

I started with baseline (before I began):

- My energy level (1–10 scale)
- My sleep quality (1–10 scale)
- My mental clarity (1–10 scale)
- My mood (1–10 scale)
- My physical capacity/limitations
- My weight
- Any disease markers if I had medical conditions

I tracked periodically (monthly or quarterly):

- My energy level (1–10 scale)
- My sleep quality (1–10 scale)
- My mental clarity (1–10 scale)
- My mood (1–10 scale)
- My physical capacity improvements
- My weight changes
- My disease markers (if testing)
- My other observations (cravings decreased, digestion improved, and so on)

I tracked medical markers (annually):

- My blood work if available (glucose, cholesterol, inflammation markers, kidney function, liver function)
- My blood pressure
- My weight and body composition
- My physical performance metrics (how far can I walk/run, how much can I lift, and so on)

Documentation proved my transformation to myself and others. It's undeniable data because after six months, I said, "I feel better," and then after 6 months with documentation, I had "energy improved from 4/10 to 8/10, sleep quality from 3/10 to 9/10, triglycerides dropped from 250 to 120."

Documentation transforms hope into evidence.

THE MOST IMPORTANT REAL-WORLD PRINCIPLE

"Raw first—not perfection"

This principle enabled my real-world transformation because it's flexible enough to sustain through real-world circumstances.

If the principle was "perfect raw food always":

- First disruption would feel like failure
- Second disruption would feel like confirmation that you can't do it
- You'd quit

But the principle is "raw first, not perfection":

- First disruption: You return to raw first, not perfectly
- Second disruption: Same response, same flexibility
- Sustainability: You keep going because the principle allows for real life

This is why I sustained for sixteen years.

Real-World Success Stories (The Pattern)

While this manifesto doesn't have other documented cases, the pattern of real-world success is:

Person X:

- Made a decision
- Started with "raw first—not perfection"
- Navigated real-world obstacles
- Documented improvements
- Over months/years: undeniable transformation
- Energy increased, health improved, capacity expanded

The specifics vary (job, family, circumstances), but the pattern is consistent.
You can be Person X.

Your circumstances are different from mine. But the principles work in *any* circumstance:

1. Make a decision
2. Implement "raw first—not perfection"

3. Navigate real-world obstacles
4. Document improvements
5. Sustain the protocol
6. Experience transformation

THE TRANSFORMATION TIMELINE: WHAT TO EXPECT

Real-world transformations follow rough timelines:

Week 1–4: Adjustment phase

- Cravings may be strong
- Energy might dip initially (withdrawal)
- Sleep might be disrupted
- By Week 4: Usually feel improvement

Month 2–3: Rapid improvement phase

- Energy noticeably improved
- Sleep quality improved
- Mental clarity improving
- Cravings decreasing
- First significant victories

Month 4–12: Sustained improvement phase

- Changes feel normal now
- Deepening of improvements
- Protocol becoming automatic
- Noticing improvements in unexpected areas (mood, capacity, and so on)

Year 2+: Long-term transformation phase

- Undeniable transformation
- Health markers significantly improved
- Capacity/vitality noticeably better
- Confidence that this is sustainable
- Inspiration to continue

Important note: Timeline varies by person. This is approximate. Patience is essential.

Real-World Measurement: Beyond the Scale

Don't measure transformation *only* by weight. Look at:

- **Energy:** "I have energy for my day" or "I need less caffeine"

- **Sleep:** "I sleep better" or "I wake feeling rested"
- **Mood:** "I feel more stable" or "I'm less anxious"
- **Capacity:** "I can do more than I could" or "Exercise feels easier"
- **Clarity:** "My thinking is clearer" or "I can concentrate better"
- **:** "I don't crave junk food" or "My hunger is stable"
- **Appearance:** "My skin looks better" or "I look healthier"
- **Clothes fit:** "My pants are looser" or "I need smaller sizes"
- **Medical markers:** "My blood pressure improved" or "My glucose is better"
- **Quality of life:** "I feel better than I have in years"

These are your *real* measurements. Not scale weight, but actual lived improvements.

How to Share Your Transformation

When your transformation is documented, it becomes powerful.
Share with:

- Your health care providers (validate your approach)
- Your family members (inspire them)
- Your friends (give them permission to consider change)
- Your community (contribute to collective understanding)

How to share:

- Humbly ("This is what worked for me")
- Factually ("Here's what I did, here's what changed")
- Without preaching ("I'm sharing, not prescribing")
- With invitation ("You could try this if it interests you")

Why share:

- Your transformation is permission for others
- Your documented data is proof of possibility
- Your story inspires others to consider change
- Collective transformation creates cultural shift

The Most Important Real-World Insight

Real transformation doesn't require:

- Perfect circumstances
- Perfect genetics
- Perfect willpower
- Perfect protocol adherence
- Other people's approval

Real transformation requires:

- A decision ("raw first—not perfection" principle)
- Navigation of real obstacles
- Consistency over time
- Self-compassion and flexibility

You have everything you need to create your transformation. The question is: will you decide?

YOUR INVITATION

You are not me. Your life is different. Your circumstances are different. Your obstacles are different.

But the principles work for *you* too.

If you:

1. Make a decision (aligned with your values)
2. Implement "raw first—not perfection" (flexibility + direction)
3. Navigate real obstacles (with compassion and adaptation)
4. Document your progress (track improvements)
5. Find community support (people who understand)
6. Sustain commitment (16 years proves it's worthwhile)

Then you will create your own documented transformation.

Not my transformation. *Your* transformation.

Based on your real life, your real circumstances, your real body, your real needs.

The Closing: Reality

This chapter is short on case studies and long on principles because the real transformation happens in *your* life, not in stories about other people.

Your transformation is the story. Your documented data is the proof. Your lived experience is the evidence.

This manifesto has given you the framework. It's shown you what's possible (my sixteen-year journey). It's provided the principles ("raw first—not perfection").

Now it's your turn.

Create your own documented transformation. In your real life. With your real circumstances. Over your own timeline.

Not perfect. But real.

Not theoretical. But actually.

Not someone else's story. But *your* story.

Your Transformation and Integration

Applying the Protocol to Your Life, Your Circumstances, Your Future

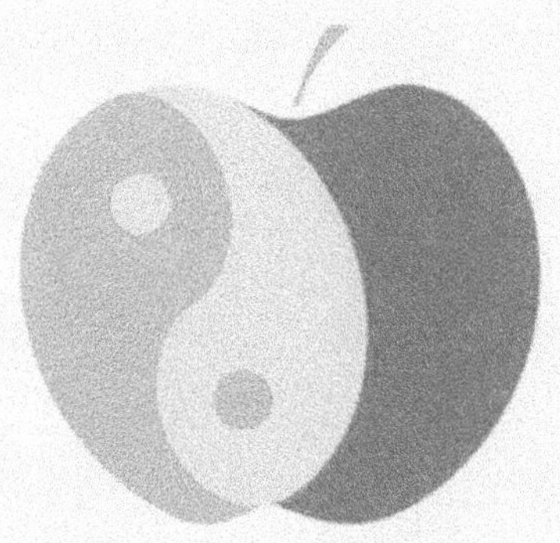

17

SPECIAL POPULATIONS

Tailored Implementation of the Energy Restoration Protocol Across Diverse Circumstances and Life Stages

ONE PROTOCOL, INFINITE ADAPTATION

The Energy Restoration Protocol is built on a unified framework: restore energy production, reduce inflammation, optimize metabolism, provide abundant micronutrients. This framework applies universally. Energy system dysfunction is the root cause of disease across all populations and life stages.

However, the specific implementation requires adaptation for different populations. A pregnant woman's nutritional needs differ from a teenager's. An elite athlete's energy demands differ from an elderly person's. A person with severe food allergies needs different food choices than someone without allergies.

This chapter provides detailed guidance for implementing the Energy Restoration Protocol across diverse special populations. The goal is not to create population-specific "diets." The goal is to maintain the core framework of whole foods, plant-based, raw when possible, no refined carbohydrates or extracted oils while adapting for each population's specific circumstances and needs.

SPECIAL POPULATION 1: PREGNANT AND BREASTFEEDING WOMEN

The Unique Circumstances

Pregnancy and breastfeeding create extraordinary nutritional demands. The pregnant woman is not just feeding herself; she's building an entire new human. The breastfeeding woman is producing food (breast milk) for an infant.

During pregnancy:

- Caloric needs increase by approximately 300–500 calories per day (second and third trimesters)
- Protein needs increase by approximately 25 grams per day
- Micronutrient needs increase dramatically: folate (to prevent neural tube defects), iron (to support expanded blood volume), calcium (for fetal bone development), DHA (for fetal brain development)
- Weight gain of twenty-five to thirty-five pounds is expected and healthy
- Energy demands are significant

During breastfeeding:

- Caloric needs increase by approximately 500 calories per day
- Protein needs remain elevated
- Micronutrient needs remain high (calcium, iron, and so on)
- Adequate hydration is critical

Protocol Adaptation for Pregnancy and Breastfeeding

The Energy Restoration Protocol remains the framework. The adaptation focuses on ensuring adequate calories, protein, and critical micronutrients.

Rather than restricting calories (which would be contraindicated during pregnancy), pregnant women on the protocol focus on eating adequate whole foods to meet their increased energy needs. This typically means:

- Eating three substantial meals plus two to three snacks daily
- Including calorie-dense foods like nuts, seeds, avocados, legumes, whole grains
- Not restricting food; eating to satisfy hunger
- Expecting and allowing appropriate weight gain

Plant-based sources of complete protein are emphasized:

- Legumes (beans, lentils, chickpeas): 15–20 grams protein per cooked cup
- Whole grains (quinoa, brown rice, oats): 5–10 grams protein per cooked cup
- Nuts and seeds (almonds, walnuts, hemp seeds, pumpkin seeds): 5–10 grams protein per ounce
- Tofu and tempeh (if tolerated): 15–20 grams protein per serving

A pregnant woman eating three meals plus snacks with these foods typically achieves adequate protein (60–70 grams daily, which is the increased recommendation during pregnancy).

Critical Micronutrients:

Folate (for neural tube development):

- Abundant in: dark leafy greens (spinach, kale), legumes, asparagus, broccoli, avocado
- Recommendation: 600 mcg daily during pregnancy (up from 400 mcg)
- Consider: a prenatal vitamin with folate for assurance, though food sources are generally adequate

Iron (for expanded blood volume):

- Abundant in: legumes, fortified grains, dark leafy greens, dried fruit (particularly raisins and apricots)
- Recommendation: 27 mg daily during pregnancy
- Enhancement: consume iron-rich foods with vitamin C (citrus, tomatoes) to enhance absorption
- Note: Plant-based iron (non-heme iron) is less bioavailable than animal iron, but adequate plant-based iron can be achieved through varied sources and vitamin C enhancement
- Consider iron supplementation if blood tests show low iron, though many pregnant women on the protocol maintain adequate iron

Calcium (for fetal bone development):

- Abundant in: leafy greens (particularly kale, collard greens, bok choy), legumes, fortified plant-based milks, tahini, tofu (if prepared with calcium)
- Recommendation: 1000–1200 mg daily
- Note: Several servings of calcium-rich plant foods daily typically provide adequate calcium

DHA (for fetal brain development):

- Abundant in: algae-based sources (spirulina, chlorella), ground flaxseeds, chia seeds, walnuts
- Recommendation: 300 mg daily during pregnancy
- Note: The body converts ALA (alpha-linolenic acid, from flaxseeds, chia, walnuts) to DHA, though conversion efficiency is variable
- Consider an algae-based DHA supplement during pregnancy and breastfeeding for assurance

Vitamin B12 (critical for pregnancy outcomes):

- Note: B12 is not naturally abundant in plant foods

- Recommendation: Nutritional Yeast Flakes, B12 supplementation or consumption of B12-fortified foods during pregnancy and breastfeeding
- This is a non-negotiable recommendation for plant-based pregnant women

Pregnant women implementing the protocol should:

- Work with an obstetrician familiar with plant-based pregnancy (midwives or OBGYNs in practice areas with higher plant-based populations are often familiar)
- Have regular blood work to monitor key markers: hemoglobin/hematocrit (for anemia), glucose (for gestational diabetes), protein (for preeclampsia risk)
- Discuss any concerns about nutrition with their health care provider
- Take prenatal vitamins as recommended by their provider

Timeline and Outcomes for Pregnant Women on the Protocol

Women implementing the protocol before pregnancy benefit from optimized health, including normal weight, optimal glucose control, and optimal micronutrient status. These factors support optimal pregnancy outcomes.

First Trimester:

- Morning sickness (if present) may be reduced due to stable blood glucose and optimized nutrient status
- Energy may improve (though fatigue in first trimester is normal)
- Weight gain is expected; no restriction
- Healthy placentation and early fetal development supported by abundant nutrients

Second and Third Trimesters:

- Gestational diabetes risk is reduced due to optimal glucose metabolism
- Preeclampsia risk is reduced due to adequate mineral intake and inflammation control
- Fetal growth is supported by adequate calories and micronutrients
- Weight gain continues (twenty-five to thirty-five pounds total is expected)
- Maternal health is maintained; energy is good

Postpartum:

- Recovery from delivery is supported by abundant nutrition
- Breastfeeding is established with adequate calories and nutrients
- Maternal weight normalization occurs naturally over months as breastfeeding continues; no restriction needed
- Emotional health is supported by stable nutrition and brain health

Infant Outcomes:

- Infants born to mothers on the protocol are typically healthy with normal birth weights and scores
- Breast milk is nutritionally adequate (though maternal B12 and DHA status should be ensured)
- Infants exposed to plant-based foods through breast milk and early introduction to foods have no increased risk; some evidence suggests reduced allergies due to diverse plant compounds in breast milk

SPECIAL POPULATION 2: CHILDREN AND ADOLESCENTS

The Unique Circumstances

Children and adolescents have different nutritional needs and developmental stages than adults. Additionally, children and adolescents are often under significant influence from school environments, peer cultures, and family food traditions.

Nutritional considerations:

- **Children (ages 4–8):** Growth is still occurring. Caloric needs are lower than adolescents but higher per pound of body weight than adults. Bone development is ongoing.
- **Preadolescents (ages 9–13):** Growth accelerates. Calcium needs to increase for bone development. Iron needs increase (particularly girls after menarche).
- **Adolescents (ages 14–18):** Growth spurt is most intense. Caloric and protein needs are elevated. Calcium, iron, and other minerals are critical for bone development.

Environmental considerations:

- **School food environments:** Most schools serve processed foods. Children may face peer pressure to eat differently from their peers.
- **Social food culture:** Food is social. Restricting children from all "normal" foods can create isolation or unhealthy relationships with food.
- **Family food traditions:** Children are learning from their family's food patterns.

Protocol Adaptation for Children and Adolescents

The protocol for children and adolescents focuses on providing abundant whole plant-based foods while allowing flexibility for social and cultural food participation. The goal is not perfect adherence but creating a strong foundation of health through optimal foods at home while allowing some social flexibility.

At home (parent-controlled):

- Meals are whole foods, plant-based, following the protocol fully
- Snacks are whole foods: fruits, vegetables, nuts, seeds
- No refined carbohydrates in the regular food supply
- No processed foods stocked at home
- This creates a strong foundation; children growing up with this as their daily food baseline are establishing healthy eating patterns

Away from home (school, social settings):

- Children are taught about the protocol and why it matters
- They're allowed to make choices at school and social settings
- The goal is not restriction but education and autonomy
- Most children, having eaten well at home, naturally make relatively good choices at school

Age-Specific Adaptations:

Children (ages four to eight):

- Meals are provided by parents/caregivers (less autonomy)
- Protocol is implemented fully at home
- Foods are presented attractively and the child is allowed to decide portion size
- Children this age, growing up with whole foods as normal, rarely have issues; they eat what's available
- School lunch: pack a protocol-compliant lunch to ensure optimal nutrition during school day

Preadolescents (ages nine to thirteen):

- Begin teaching understanding of *why* the protocol matters
- Children have increasing autonomy in food choices
- At home: protocol is maintained
- At school: children navigate school lunches; many pack protocol-compliant lunches
- Social settings: children are taught to make good choices while allowing some flexibility
- Peer influence becomes stronger; parents support children in navigating this

Adolescents (ages fourteen to eighteen):

- Full explanation of the protocol and the science behind it
- Adolescents have autonomy in food choices, with parental guidance
- Many adolescents, understanding the connection between food and how they feel, maintain protocol adherence voluntarily

- Some adolescents experiment with other foods at social settings; this is normal and expected
- The foundation of health established in childhood supports good choices even with some social flexibility

The most common challenge for children and adolescents on the protocol is social pressure. Friends eating different foods, school lunches, birthday parties, social gatherings all present situations where the child is different from their peers.

The approach:

1. **Don't make it a statement.** The goal is not for the child to be the conscious objector or to make others feel judged. It's just what they eat.
2. **Allow flexibility.** Most successful families allow children to make some choices at social settings. Rigid restriction creates rebellion or unhealthy relationships with food.
3. **Focus on health, not rules.** Children who understand that the protocol helps them feel better, have more energy, think more clearly, perform better athletically and academically are more likely to choose it voluntarily.
4. **Be present.** Parents modeling protocol adherence and living it themselves is far more powerful than rules imposed on children.

Specific Nutritional Considerations:

Calcium for growing bones:

- Adequate sources: fortified plant-based milks, leafy greens, legumes, tahini, tofu
- Recommendation: 1000–1300 mg daily for growing children and adolescents
- Ensure adequate intake through food or fortified plant-based milk

Iron for adolescent girls:

- Increased needs for menstruating girls (18 mg daily vs. 11 mg for boys)
- Abundant sources: legumes, fortified grains, leafy greens, dried fruit
- Enhance absorption with vitamin C
- Monitor via blood work if concerned about iron status

Protein for growth:

- Adequate sources: legumes, whole grains, nuts, seeds
- Recommendation: 0.85–1.0 grams per pound of body weight (varies by age)
- Most children eating three meals plus snacks with these foods achieve adequate protein

Timeline and Outcomes for Children and Adolescents on the Protocol

Childhood (ages four to eight):

- Children growing up with whole foods as their baseline eat protocol foods naturally
- Energy and athletic capacity are often above average
- Academic performance is often strong (brain receiving optimal nutrition and energy)
- Weight is healthy; childhood obesity is prevented
- Chronic health issues (allergies, asthma, eczema) often improve or resolve
- Children have strong immune function; fewer colds and infections

Preadolescence (ages nine to thirteen):

- As peers increasingly consume processed foods, children may question their eating
- Schools increasingly influence diet (school lunches, peer food culture)
- Most children, if they understand why the protocol matters and if parents maintain family support, continue it
- Some children experiment with other foods at social settings; this is normal
- Physical capacity, athletic performance, academic performance remain strong
- Emotional stability is typically good (compared to peers experiencing blood sugar dysregulation)

Adolescence (ages fourteen to eighteen):

- Adolescents have more autonomy and often more social pressure to conform to peer eating
- Adolescents who understand the connection between food and energy/mood/performance often maintain the protocol voluntarily
- Many adolescents benefit from explicit teaching about the protocol: why it matters, how it works, what choices are available to them
- Skin (often a concern for adolescents) is typically clear on the protocol, which many adolescents find motivating
- Energy, focus, and athletic/academic performance are typically excellent
- Some adolescents experiment with other foods; this experimentation is normal and often temporary
- Most adolescents who grew up with the protocol maintain it into adulthood, though some take breaks and return to it

Young adulthood (ages eighteen and over):

- Young adults who grew up on the protocol typically maintain it voluntarily
- Many have tried other eating patterns and returned to the protocol because of how much better they feel on it
- These young adults, having established the protocol as their baseline, pass it to their own children
- Multigenerational health benefit: parents on the protocol, children on the protocol, grandchildren on the protocol

SPECIAL POPULATION 3: ATHLETES

Athletic performance creates high energy demands. Additionally, athletes often face beliefs about what they need to eat for performance (often emphasizing animal protein and specific sports supplements).

Energy considerations:

- Endurance athletes: Extremely high caloric needs; can require 4000–6000+ calories daily
- Strength athletes: High-protein needs and high-caloric needs; can require 3000–5000+ calories daily
- High-intensity athletes: High-carbohydrate needs for glycogen replenishment; moderate-high-caloric needs

Misconceptions:

- "Athletes need animal protein" (plant-based protein is equally effective)
- "Athletes need refined carbohydrates" (whole carbohydrates perform equally well)
- "Athletes need special supplements" (whole foods typically provide all needed nutrients)
- "Plant-based athletes have lower performance" (elite plant-based athletes consistently perform at high levels)

Protocol Adaptation for Athletes

The Energy Restoration Protocol is actually optimal for athletic performance. The abundant whole plant foods provide both the energy and the micronutrients needed for optimal performance and recovery.

Rather than counting calories or macronutrients obsessively, athletes on the protocol focus on eating abundant whole foods to meet their energy needs. Most athletes eating three to four substantial meals plus two to three snacks of whole plant foods naturally achieve the calories and macronutrients they need.

Energy and caloric adequacy:

Athletes implement the protocol exactly as described, but with emphasis on adequate total calories:

- Eat to satisfaction; don't restrict
- Include calorie-dense whole foods: nuts, seeds, legumes, whole grains, avocados, olive oil (in moderation, but used)
- Eat frequent meals and snacks
- Monitor energy levels; if energy drops, eat more

A typical athlete might eat:

- Breakfast: Oatmeal with banana and nuts, plus toast with almond butter (600+ calories)
- Midmorning snack: Fruit and nuts (200–300 calories)
- Lunch: Fruits, Large salad, whole grains, vegetables, nuts (600–800 calories)
- Afternoon snack: Whole grain crackers with hummus (300–400 calories)
- Dinner: Legumes, whole grains, large vegetable portion, nuts/seeds (700–900 calories)
- Evening snack (if desired): vegetables and nuts (200–300 calories)

Total: 3000–4300 calories, exactly what many athletes need.

Protein for athletic performance:

Plant-based proteins support athletic performance equally to animal proteins. Athletes on the protocol achieve adequate protein through:

- Legumes: 15–20 grams per cooked cup
- Whole grains (particularly quinoa): 5–10 grams per cooked cup
- Nuts and seeds: 5–10 grams per ounce
- Multiple servings throughout the day naturally accumulating to 60–100+ grams daily, depending on the athlete's needs

An athlete eating three meals plus snacks with these foods typically achieves optimal protein intake.

Carbohydrates for energy and recovery:

Whole carbohydrates (legumes, whole grains, fruits, vegetables) provide the energy athletes need for performance and the glycogen replenishment they need for recovery.

- Whole grains: 30–40 grams carbohydrate per cooked cup
- Legumes: 30–40 grams carbohydrate per cooked cup

- Fruits: 25–35 grams carbohydrate each
- Multiple servings throughout the day provide abundant carbohydrates

Endurance athletes particularly benefit from the glycogen stores provided by these foods.

Micronutrients for performance and recovery:

The abundant plant foods provide:

- Antioxidants for managing exercise-induced oxidative stress
- Minerals (magnesium, potassium, iron, zinc) for muscle function and recovery
- B vitamins for energy metabolism
- Anti-inflammatory compounds for managing inflammation from intense training

Hydration and electrolytes:

Athletes on the protocol maintain hydration through:

- Adequate water intake
- Electrolytes from whole foods: potassium from legumes, fruits; magnesium from leafy greens; sodium from sea salt in cooking

Most athletes find this adequate without specialized sports drinks.

Timing around training:

- Pre-exercise meal: Eaten two to three hours before training; substantial meal with carbohydrates and protein
- Post-exercise meal/snack: Eaten within one to two hours after training; meal with carbohydrates and protein to replenish glycogen and support muscle recovery

Special considerations for different types of athletes:

Endurance athletes (marathoners, distance runners, cyclists, triathletes):

- Very high caloric needs (4000–6000+ calories daily for some athletes)
- Emphasis on abundant whole grains, legumes, and carbohydrate-rich foods
- Adequate B vitamins for energy metabolism
- Iron-rich foods with vitamin C for enhanced absorption
- Example: An ultramarathon runner on the protocol eats 4000–5000 calories daily from whole foods, experiences high-level performance, and recovers well

Strength athletes (weightlifters, bodybuilders, football players):

- High protein needs (60–100+ grams daily)

- Caloric surplus for muscle building
- Adequate energy through carbohydrates for training intensity
- Legumes, nuts, seeds, and whole grains provide adequate protein
- Example: A bodybuilder on the protocol builds muscle effectively on plant-based protein; body composition is excellent

High-intensity athletes (sprinters, crossfitters, basketball players):

- High energy needs for intense training
- Abundant carbohydrates for glycogen replenishment between sets/matches
- Adequate protein for muscle recovery
- Whole foods provide all needed nutrients
- Example: A CrossFit athlete on the protocol performs at elite levels with whole food fueling

Timeline and Outcomes for Athletes on the Protocol

Initial implementation (Weeks 1–4):

- Energy may initially feel slightly different as glycogen replenishment switches from refined carbs to whole carbs
- Most athletes adapt within one to two weeks
- Performance typically improves as inflammation decreases and mitochondrial efficiency increases

Adaptation phase (Months 1–3):

- Athletic performance improves; strength and endurance increase
- Recovery improves; athletes feel less sore, bounce back faster
- Body composition often improves
- Motivation and mental clarity improve
- Sleep quality improves

Optimization phase (Month 3+):

- Peak performance is typically achieved
- Athletes report "feeling better than ever"
- Injury rate decreases due to anti-inflammatory eating
- Consistency is excellent; athletes maintain training without illness-related absences
- Career longevity is often extended (many plant-based athletes have longer careers than their processed-food-consuming peers)

SPECIAL POPULATION 4: SENIORS (OVER SIXTY-FIVE)

The Unique Circumstances

Seniors face specific health challenges and needs:

- Cognitive function: Prevention or slowing of cognitive decline is paramount
- Physical capacity: Maintaining strength and mobility is critical for independence
- Bone health: Bone density naturally decreases; maintaining adequate calcium and magnesium is important
- Chronic disease prevalence: Seniors often have multiple conditions
- Medication complexity: Seniors often take multiple medications with potential interactions
- Nutritional absorption: Stomach acid and digestive function may be reduced

Protocol Adaptation for Seniors

The Energy Restoration Protocol is remarkably beneficial for seniors. By restoring energy production and reducing inflammation, the protocol supports cognitive maintenance, physical capacity preservation, and chronic disease prevention or reversal.

Seniors implement the protocol as described, with attention to adequate protein and micronutrients:

Protein for muscle maintenance:

Seniors need adequate protein to maintain muscle mass (which naturally declines with age). Plant-based sources provide adequate protein:

- Legumes: 15–20 grams per cooked cup
- Whole grains: 5–10 grams per cooked cup
- Nuts and seeds: 5–10 grams per ounce
- Recommendation: 1.0–1.2 grams per kilogram of body weight daily

Most seniors eating three meals plus snacks with these foods achieve adequate protein.

Micronutrients for Bone and Cognitive Health:

Calcium for bone density:

- Abundant sources: leafy greens (particularly kale, collard greens), fortified plant-based milks, legumes, tahini
- Recommendation: 1000–1200 mg daily

- Consider: strength training (weight-bearing exercise) maintains bone density as effectively as calcium alone
- Magnesium for bone and cognitive health:
- Abundant sources: leafy greens, legumes, seeds, nuts, whole grains
- Recommendation: 400–420 mg daily for men, 310–320 mg daily for women
- Research: magnesium has been shown to support cognitive function and reduce cognitive decline risk

Vitamin B12 for cognitive health:

- Non-negotiable: B12 supplementation or fortified foods
- B12 deficiency has been linked to cognitive decline and increased dementia risk
- Plant-based seniors should ensure adequate B12

Omega-3 fatty acids (ALA and DHA) for cognitive health:

- Abundant sources: flaxseeds, chia seeds, walnuts, leafy greens
- Consider: algae-based DHA supplement if concerned about conversion
- Research: adequate omega-3 intake has been associated with cognitive preservation

Managing chronic conditions:

Seniors implementing the protocol often have existing chronic conditions (diabetes, hypertension, cardiovascular disease, arthritis, cognitive impairment). The protocol supports:

- Reversal of some conditions (particularly metabolic diseases like diabetes and hypertension)
- Stabilization of progressive conditions
- Prevention of new condition development

Medical coordination is important; medications may need adjustment as health improves.

Cognitive function preservation and improvement:

One of the most striking benefits for seniors is cognitive preservation and often improvement. The protocol supports brain health through:

- Abundant energy production in brain cells
- Reduction of neuroinflammation
- Abundant antioxidants protecting brain tissue

- Stable blood glucose preventing neurotoxic effects of dysregulation
- Adequate micronutrients supporting neurotransmitter production

Many seniors report that their cognitive function improves on the protocol; they become sharper and more mentally capable than they were in previous years.

Physical capacity preservation:

Adequate protein and the anti-inflammatory effects of the protocol support physical capacity preservation:

- Strength is maintained with adequate protein and resistance training
- Flexibility is maintained with physical activity
- Endurance is maintained with aerobic activity
- Joint health is supported by reduced inflammation

Many seniors on the protocol maintain athletic capacity: running, hiking, yoga, strength training well into advanced age.

Medication interactions and medical coordination:

Seniors taking medications should:

- Work with their doctor as health improves and medications may need adjustment
- Ensure health care provider knows about dietary changes
- Coordinate any supplement use (B12, DHA, and so on) with medications
- Have regular blood work to monitor health markers

Timeline and Outcomes for Seniors on the Protocol

Initial implementation (Weeks 1–4):

- Energy improves
- Sleep quality improves
- Digestion improves
- Mental clarity improves
- Physical capacity feels better

Adjustment phase (Months 1–3):

- Chronic conditions begin improving (if present)
- Medications may need adjustment (in coordination with health care provider)
- Cognitive function improves noticeably
- Physical capacity continues improving
- Overall vitality increases

Long-term (Month 3+):

- Cognitive function remains excellent or continues improving
- Physical capacity is maintained or continues improving
- Chronic disease is prevented, stabilized, or reversed
- Quality of life is high
- Many seniors report that they feel younger than their age

SPECIAL POPULATION 5: PEOPLE WITH LIMITED INCOME

The Unique Circumstances

Economic constraints create real food access challenges. Yet, the protocol is accessible to people with limited income through strategic, creative implementation.

Economic realities:

- Budget constraints: Limited money for food
- Food desert realities: Limited access to fresh produce
- Time constraints: Limited time for food preparation
- Food access limitations: Limited food storage (refrigeration, freezing)

Protocol Adaptation for Limited-Income Populations

The protocol is actually economically accessible because whole foods are cheaper than processed foods when purchased unprocessed.

Budget strategy:

- Buy in bulk: Dried beans, lentils, rice, oats, nuts are cheapest when bought from bulk bins
- Seasonal produce: Buying seasonal produce is much cheaper than out-of-season
- Frozen vegetables: Often cheaper than fresh and equally nutritious; reduces food waste
- Canned vegetables and beans: Affordable and convenient; canned is better than processed
- Discounted stores: Walmart, discount grocers, food co-ops offer affordable options
- Community resources: Food banks, community gardens, farmer's market sales often provide affordable produce

Budget meals:

Meals can be protocol-compliant and extremely affordable:

- Breakfast: Oatmeal with banana and peanuts (~$1)

- Lunch: Bean soup with vegetables (~$1.50)
- Dinner: Rice and beans with canned vegetables (~$1.50)
- Snacks: Apples, bananas, peanuts (~$1)

Total: ~$5 daily, well within limited budgets.

Time and resource constraints:

Limited time can be addressed through:

- Batch cooking: Making large pots of soup, chili, legume dishes on weekends
- Simple meals: Not requiring complex recipes; basic combinations of legumes, grains, vegetables
- Minimal cooking: Some meals require minimal cooking (whole grain with canned beans, fresh vegetables)

Limited food storage can be addressed through:

- Shelf-stable whole foods: Beans, lentils, rice, oats, canned vegetables don't require refrigeration
- Minimal fresh produce: Buying small amounts of fresh produce as needed rather than large quantities
- Frozen vegetables: Take up freezer space but don't require fresh produce access

Special Resources for Limited-Income Implementation

- Food banks: Often have canned beans, vegetables, grains available
- Community gardens: Many communities have gardens where residents can grow vegetables for free or minimal cost
- Farmer's market discounts: Some markets have free produce for low-income individuals, or discounted prices for seniors
- SNAP benefits (food stamps): All the whole foods recommended in the protocol qualify for SNAP
- Community organizations: Churches, nonprofits, community centers often provide resources for limited-income populations

Mindset Shift for Limited-Income Implementation

The critical mindset shift is understanding that *you don't need to be wealthy to eat well.* The processed food industry has positioned expensive specialty foods and restaurants as healthy. In reality, the cheapest, healthiest foods are whole plant foods bought unprocessed.

SPECIAL POPULATION 6: PEOPLE WITH FOOD ALLERGIES OR INTOLERANCES

The Unique Circumstances

Severe food allergies (peanuts, tree nuts, soy, shellfish, and so on) or intolerances (gluten, certain legumes, and so on) create constraints on food choices.

The protocol is flexible enough to work with most allergies and intolerances, though specific adaptations are needed.

Protocol Adaptation for Allergies and Intolerances

Nut/peanut allergies:

If unable to eat nuts or seeds:

- Emphasize legumes (beans, lentils, chickpeas), whole grains, avocado for healthy fats. Legumes provide protein and healthy fats previously provided by nuts.
- Olive oil (used in moderation, primarily for flavor) can provide additional fat-soluble nutrients

Soy allergies:

If unable to eat soy (tofu, tempeh):

- Emphasize other legumes (beans, lentils, chickpeas), nuts, seeds, whole grains
- No significant limitation; many plant-based proteins available without soy

Gluten sensitivity/celiac disease:

If unable to eat wheat/gluten:

- Emphasize rice, quinoa, potatoes, oats (gluten-free), legumes, vegetables, fruits
- Abundant gluten-free whole grains and foods available
- No significant limitation to protocol

Legume intolerances:

If unable to eat legumes (beans, lentils, chickpeas):

- More challenging, as legumes are protein-rich
- Compensate with abundant nuts, seeds, whole grains (particularly quinoa), avocado
- Requires careful attention to protein adequacy
- May benefit from working with a dietitian to ensure adequate nutrition

Multiple allergies:

If multiple allergies are present:

- Case-by-case adaptation needed
- Work with a dietitian familiar with plant-based eating to ensure adequate nutrition
- The protocol's core principle (whole foods, plant-based, emphasis on vegetables and legumes) remains valid; specific foods are adapted

SPECIAL POPULATION 7: PEOPLE WITH SEVERE MENTAL ILLNESS

The Unique Circumstances

Severe mental illnesses (schizophrenia, bipolar disorder, severe depression) often require psychiatric medication management. The Energy Restoration Protocol supports psychiatric medication effectiveness and can enable medication reduction, but medication should not be discontinued without psychiatric supervision.

Additionally, psychiatric conditions may make dietary adherence challenging (lack of motivation, cognitive impairment, medication side effects affecting appetite or food preferences).

Protocol Adaptation for Severe Mental Illness

The protocol supports psychiatric treatment by:

- Providing optimal brain nutrition and energy
- Reducing neuroinflammation
- Stabilizing blood glucose (affecting mood and cognitive function)
- Supporting medication effectiveness

Psychiatric medications remain important. The protocol is supplementary, not a replacement.

Implementation approach:

- Psychiatric coordination is essential: Health care provider should know about dietary changes; medication adjustments may be needed as health improves.
- Start gradually: For people with significant psychiatric symptoms, starting suddenly with major dietary change may be destabilizing. Gradual implementation is often better.
- Support systems are important: Family support, care team support, mental health professional support all help adherence.
- Medication stability first: In acute crises, medication management comes first. Dietary change can follow stabilization.

- Long-term benefit: As psychiatric stability is achieved through medication, adding the protocol often provides additional benefit as it can improve energy, improve mood stability, improve cognitive function, reduce medication side effects.

Special considerations:

- Medication side effects: Some psychiatric medications affect appetite or food preferences. Address with a health care provider.
- Motivation and executive function: Some psychiatric conditions impair motivation and executive function, making meal planning and cooking challenging. Simplify recipes, use batch cooking, consider ready-to-eat protocol foods.
- Food preparation: If cognitive or motivational impairment makes cooking difficult, emphasize easy options: canned beans, frozen vegetables, simple combinations requiring minimal cooking.

ADDITIONAL SPECIAL POPULATIONS

The above populations represent major life stages and circumstances. Additional special populations where the protocol is beneficial include:

People with food addictions/compulsive eating: The protocol, providing stable blood glucose and abundant nutrition, supports recovery from food addiction. As cravings resolve and appetite normalizes, recovery becomes sustainable.

People with eating disorders (in recovery): The protocol, providing abundant nutrition and normal eating patterns, supports recovery. Should be implemented under professional supervision (therapist and/or dietitian specializing in eating disorders).

Autistic individuals: Some autistic individuals have sensory sensitivities or rigid food preferences that make protocol implementation challenging. However, many autistic individuals thrive on the protocol once implementation is adapted for sensory preferences. Individualized approach needed.

People with diabetes-related kidney disease: The protocol can be implemented but requires medical coordination regarding protein intake and mineral balance. Significant health improvements are possible.

People with autoimmune conditions: The protocol's anti-inflammatory approach often significantly improves autoimmune conditions. Implementation should be coordinated with rheumatologist or other specialist.

The Unifying Principle: Adaptation, Not Abandonment

The central principle across all special populations is that the Energy Restoration Protocol adapts to circumstances; circumstances don't prevent implementation.

The core framework remains consistent: whole foods, plant-based, abundant micronutrients, no refined carbohydrates, no extracted oils, no processed foods.

The specific implementation adapts to each population's unique needs, circumstances, and constraints.

A pregnant woman, a teenager, an elite athlete, an elderly person, someone living in poverty, someone with food allergies all can implement the protocol. The framework is consistent. The adaptation is specific.

This is the power and the elegance of the protocol: universal principle, infinite adaptation.

Moving Forward

These special population adaptations demonstrate that the Energy Restoration Protocol is not a one-size-fits-all approach that works only in ideal circumstances. It's a flexible framework that adapts to diverse populations, circumstances, and life stages.

The next chapter, "Long-Term Sustainability," explores how people maintain the protocol indefinitely and specifically addresses movement and exercise integration and how physical activity synergizes with the protocol for optimal health throughout life.

18

LONG-TERM SUSTAINABILITY

How to Maintain the Energy Restoration Protocol and Integrate Movement for Lifelong Health

SUSTAINABILITY IS THE ENTIRE POINT

Throughout this manifesto, we've explored the Energy Restoration Protocol's remarkable ability to reverse disease, prevent disease, and optimize health. But there's a critical distinction between temporary improvement and sustained transformation.

Temporary improvement is when a person implements the protocol, sees dramatic health benefits for six to twelve months, then gradually returns to previous patterns as motivation wanes, circumstances change, or old habits reassert. The improvements fade. The disease often returns.

Sustained transformation is when a person implements the protocol, sees dramatic health benefits, and continues the protocol indefinitely because it becomes their normal way of living. The improvements are permanent. The disease doesn't return. Health continues optimizing across decades.

This chapter addresses sustained transformation: how people maintain the protocol long-term, how movement and exercise integrate with the protocol for maximum benefit, and how to build a life where health is simply how you live, not something you have to fight for.

THE FUNDAMENTAL SHIFT: FROM "DOING A DIET" TO "LIVING A LIFE"

The most critical insight for long-term sustainability is understanding that the Energy Restoration Protocol is not a "diet." Diets are temporary interventions you "do" for a period of time. They require willpower. They're at odds with normal life. Eventually, you stop dieting and return to normal eating.

The Energy Restoration Protocol, when implemented successfully long-term, is not experienced as a diet. It's experienced as simply how you eat. It's normal. It requires no willpower because there's nothing to resist; it's just what you do.

The shift from "doing the protocol" to "living the protocol" is the shift from temporary to sustained.

What Changes from Temporary to Sustained

Initial implementation (Weeks 1–12):

- Conscious effort required
- Active decision-making about food choices
- Reliance on willpower and motivation
- Experienced as "being on" the protocol
- Results are motivating; people are excited about changes

Transition phase (Months 3–12):

- Conscious effort gradually decreases
- The protocol becomes increasingly normal
- Willpower becomes less necessary; habits are established
- People still think about the protocol, but less actively
- Results are now experienced as normal, not exceptional

Sustained phase (Year 1+):

- The protocol is simply how you eat
- No conscious effort required
- No reliance on willpower; it's automatic
- People stop thinking about "being on" the protocol; it's just eating
- Health is experienced as normal, not exceptional
- Deviation from the protocol feels unnatural (not because of restriction, but because the alternatives feel wrong)

This evolution from conscious effort to automatic habit is what enables long-term sustainability.

THE CONDITIONS FOR LONG-TERM SUSTAINABILITY

What conditions enable people to transition from conscious implementation to sustained living of the protocol? Research on habit formation and long-term behavior change suggests several factors:

Identity Integration

Long-term sustainability is most stable when the protocol becomes integrated into personal identity. Rather than "I'm following a protocol," it becomes "I'm someone who eats plant-based whole foods and takes care of my health."

Identity-based living is more stable than rule-based living because it doesn't depend on willpower or constant decision-making. It depends on how you see yourself.

How to build this:

- **Explicitly adopt the identity.** "I'm someone who eats plant-based foods." "I'm someone who prioritizes health." These statements, repeated internally and externally, gradually become integrated.
- **Align actions with identity.** Each time you choose protocol-aligned foods or actions, you strengthen the identity. Each time you deviate, you weaken it. (This doesn't mean perfectionism; it means overall pattern.)
- **Find your community.** Being around others living similarly reinforces the identity and normalizes the patterns.
- **Tell your story.** Articulating why the protocol matters to you and sharing it with others strengthens your commitment and identity.

Environmental Design

People are more likely to sustain behaviors when their environment supports them. Rather than relying on willpower to choose healthy foods in an environment full of processed foods, design an environment where healthy foods are the default.

How to build this:

- **Stock your home with protocol foods only.** If unhealthy foods aren't in your home, you won't eat them at home. You may eat them occasionally outside the home, but your baseline is set by what's available.
- **Organize your kitchen for ease.** Fresh vegetables in visible locations. Legumes and grains stored accessibly. Nuts and seeds in bowls on the counter. Making protocol-aligned eating easier than searching for alternatives.
- **Plan meal prep into your schedule.** Batch cooking on weekends becomes routine. The rhythm is established. Meals are ready during the week.
- **Reduce friction for protocol adherence.** The easier it is to stay protocol-aligned, the more likely you will.

Social Support

Long-term sustainability is significantly easier with social support. People are more likely to maintain health behaviors when others around them support it, understand it, or live similarly.

How to build this:

- **Involve family.** If family members adopt the protocol too, the whole household dynamic changes. Eating protocol foods becomes normal for everyone.
- **Build community.** Finding others living similarly through online communities, local plant-based groups, cooking classes, and so on. provides support and normalization.
- **Communicate with your health care provider.** A provider who understands and supports the protocol can remove concerns about medical complications.
- **Involve friends.** Spending time with people supportive of your lifestyle normalizes it and makes adherence easier.

System Integration

Long-term sustainability is easier when the protocol is integrated into your systems and routines, rather than something added on top of existing systems.

How to build this:

- **Integrate meal planning and prep into your schedule.** It becomes part of your weekly routine, like doing laundry.
- **Integrate movement into your daily life.** Exercise isn't something you have to force; it's woven into how you live.
- **Integrate health monitoring into your routines.** Annual checkups, blood work, tracking of health markers become part of your normal health maintenance.
- **Integrate protocol adherence into your professional and social life.** You know what to order at restaurants. You know what to say when offered food that doesn't align with the protocol.

Flexibility Without Abandonment

This is crucial: long-term sustainability requires flexibility. Perfect adherence is not sustainable. Perfect adherence requires constant vigilance and creates rigidity that eventually breaks.

What *is* sustainable is flexible adherence—you follow the protocol as your baseline (probably 90 percent of the time), but you allow flexibility in specific contexts:

- Social events where the food isn't protocol-aligned, and you want to be present with people
- Cultural celebrations involving traditional foods that matter to your heritage
- Occasional deviations that don't derail your overall pattern

Flexible adherence maintains the benefits while allowing life to be lived fully.

MOVEMENT AND EXERCISE: THE ESSENTIAL COMPLEMENT TO NUTRITION

Up to this point in the manifesto, we've focused primarily on the nutritional component of the Energy Restoration Protocol. But the protocol is not purely about food. It's about energy system restoration. Movement and exercise are integral to this restoration.

Why Movement Is Essential for Energy Production

If someone is energy-depleted, wouldn't movement deplete them further?

The reality is more nuanced—appropriate movement actually *increases* energy production and availability.

The mitochondrial response to movement:

When you exercise, you create demand for energy. Your muscles demand ATP. In response to this demand, your body upregulates mitochondrial function. Over time (days to weeks), this results in:

- Increased mitochondrial number in muscle cells
- Increased mitochondrial efficiency
- Increased ATP production capacity

This is why people often report feeling *more* energetic after starting exercise, even though exercise initially depletes energy. The adaptation to increased demand creates increased capacity.

Additionally, exercise:

- Improves insulin sensitivity: Movement improves glucose uptake and metabolic function
- Reduces inflammation: Exercise reduces systemic inflammatory markers
- Improves blood flow: Better oxygen delivery to all tissues
- Supports brain health: Exercise increases BDNF (brain-derived neurotrophic factor), supporting neural health and cognitive function
- Improves sleep: Exercise supports deep, restorative sleep
- Improves mood: Exercise increases endorphins and supports mental health

The combination of optimal nutrition *and* appropriate movement creates exponentially greater benefits than either alone.

Timeline of Exercise Tolerance During Protocol Implementation

Weeks 1–2:

- Initial exercise capacity may feel slightly different as glycogen sources shift from refined carbs to whole carbs

- Some people feel slightly fatigued initially
- Most people adapt by end of Week 2 and begin feeling better with exercise

Weeks 3–4:

- Exercise tolerance noticeably improves
- Recovery from exercise improves (less soreness, bounces back faster)
- Energy for exercise increases
- Exercise feels easier despite same intensity

Month 1–2:

- Exercise capacity substantially improves
- Strength increases
- Endurance increases
- Recovery is excellent
- Exercise is energizing rather than depleting

Month 2–6:

- Peak exercise capacity is typically achieved
- Athletic performance continues improving for athletes
- Exercise becomes a natural, energizing part of the day

Types of Movement for Energy Restoration

Different types of movement serve different purposes in the Energy Restoration framework:

Aerobic exercise (moderate-intensity sustained movement)

Examples: Walking, jogging, cycling, swimming, hiking, rowing

Duration: 150+ minutes weekly of moderate intensity, or 75+ minutes of vigorous intensity

Benefits:

- Cardiovascular health optimization
- Metabolic improvement
- Mitochondrial function optimization
- Mental health support
- Sleep improvement

Strength training (resistance-based movement)

Examples: Weight training, bodyweight exercises, resistance bands, functional movement

Duration: Two to three sessions weekly, working major muscle groups
Benefits:

- Muscle maintenance and building
- Bone health (weight-bearing)
- Metabolic health (muscle is metabolically active)
- Functional strength for daily activities
- Injury prevention

Flexibility and mobility work

Examples: Yoga, stretching, tai chi, Pilates

Duration: Two to three sessions weekly, or daily if brief

Benefits:

- Joint health and mobility
- Injury prevention
- Nervous system balance
- Mental clarity and stress reduction
- Movement quality

High-intensity interval training (HIIT)

Examples: Sprint intervals, circuit training, vigorous sport play

Duration: One to two sessions weekly, fifteen to thirty minutes

Benefits:

- Time-efficient cardiovascular improvement
- Mitochondrial function optimization (rapid ATP demand)
- Metabolic improvement
- Performance gains for athletes

Daily movement (non-exercise)

Examples: Walking, gardening, household work, recreational activities

Duration: Throughout the day, multiple short bouts

Benefits:

- Baseline activity supports health
- Reduces sedentary time
- Supports daily energy and mood
- Injury prevention from sedentary lifestyle

Recommended Movement Framework

A sustainable, comprehensive movement practice includes components of all these types:

Weekly structure (for nonathletes):

- 150+ minutes aerobic exercise (can be spread throughout week: 30 minutes x 5 days, or any distribution)
- Two to three strength training sessions (thirty to forty-five minutes each)
- Two to three flexibility/mobility sessions (twenty to thirty minutes each)
- Daily movement/activity

For athletes, intensity and duration scale according to sport and competitive demands.

Important principle: movement should feel good.

The best exercise program is one you'll actually do. This means:

- **Choose a movement you enjoy.** Someone who enjoys walking will sustain a walking program. Someone who hates running won't sustain running.
- **Build community around movement.** Exercise with others, take classes, join groups. The social component increases adherence.
- **Start with realistic expectations.** If you're sedentary, start with ten to fifteen minutes daily and build gradually. Don't start with sixty minutes daily.
- **Listen to your body.** Soreness is normal initially; pain is not. Adjust appropriately.

Exercise and the Thirty-Day Reset: Timing Considerations

For someone implementing the Energy Restoration Protocol with the thirty-day reset specifically:

Days 1–7 (adjustment phase):

- Maintain current exercise level, but don't increase intensity
- Exercise may feel slightly different as energy systems shift
- Recovery may feel slightly different; this is normal
- Listen to your body; if extreme fatigue, reduce exercise and focus on recovery

Days 8–14 (recalibration phase):

- Exercise begins feeling better
- Recovery improves noticeably
- Can maintain current exercise with confidence
- Can gradually increase intensity if desired

Days 15–30 (optimization phase):

- Exercise capacity is noticeably improved
- This is often when people feel ready to increase exercise intensity or volume
- Be cautious about overtraining; increased exercise capacity should be built gradually

Beyond thirty days:

- Exercise can be optimized and intensified according to goals
- The combination of optimal nutrition and consistent movement creates sustained health optimization

LONG-TERM MOVEMENT PRACTICE: AGE-APPROPRIATE RECOMMENDATIONS

Movement and exercise recommendations vary by age because capabilities and health considerations change:

Young Adults (Twenty to Forty)

Considerations: Peak physical capacity, building habits for life, often establishing exercise patterns that continue for decades.

Recommendations:

- Aerobic exercise: 150+ minutes weekly, can include competitive sports
- Strength training: Two to three sessions weekly; good time to build foundational strength
- Flexibility: Two to three sessions weekly
- High intensity: One to two sessions weekly (capacity is high)

Focus: Building habits, establishing sustainable practices, exploring different activities to find what you enjoy.

Middle Adults (Forty to Sixty-Five)

Considerations: Life often includes career demands, family responsibilities; movement may need to fit within constraints; this is critical period for maintaining capacity.

Recommendations:

- Aerobic exercise: 150+ minutes weekly; can include walking, cycling, recreational sports
- Strength training: Two to three sessions weekly; becomes increasingly important for maintaining muscle and bone

- Flexibility: Two to three sessions weekly; injury prevention becomes more important
- High intensity: One to two sessions weekly, scaled to individual capacity

Focus: Consistency and sustainability, building movement that fits into life, injury prevention, maintaining capacity built in younger years.

Older Adults (Over Sixty-Five)

Considerations: Maintaining independence, bone and muscle health critical, chronic conditions may be present, recovery may take longer.

Recommendations:

- Aerobic exercise: 150+ minutes weekly of moderate intensity; walking, water aerobics, cycling
- Strength training: Two to three sessions weekly; focus on functional strength and fall prevention
- Flexibility: Three to five sessions weekly; mobility and flexibility become primary focus
- Balance training: Daily or several times weekly; essential for fall prevention and independence
- Intensity: Moderate rather than high; focus on consistency and sustainability

Focus: Maintaining independence and functional capacity, fall prevention, managing chronic conditions through movement, enjoying activity for its own sake.

BUILDING YOUR OWN SUSTAINABLE PRACTICE

For anyone seeking to maintain the Energy Restoration Protocol and consistent movement long-term, specific elements support sustainability.

Make It Automatic

The more automatic your practices become, the more sustainable they are:

- Meal prep routine: Make it a scheduled part of your week (for example, Sunday afternoon), not something you have to think about.
- Exercise routine: Schedule workouts like appointments; they're non-negotiable parts of your week.
- Health monitoring: Annual checkups, blood work (make them routine)

Build in Enjoyment

Practices maintained long-term are ones that bring genuine enjoyment:

- Find foods you love: Yes, you eat healthier foods, but there are plenty you'll genuinely enjoy. Find them.

- Find movement you love: Whether running, swimming, yoga, dancing, or hiking, find what brings you joy.
- Build community: Meal prep with others, exercise with others, celebrate health together.

Track Progress Objectively

Objective measures of improvement help maintain motivation:

- Medical markers: Annual blood work showing improvements is motivating
- Performance metrics: Faster running times, increased strength, better flexibility
- How you feel: Energy levels, sleep quality, mood stability all objectively better
- Visible progress: Body composition, appearance often improving

Adjust as Life Changes

Life changes: work demands shift, family situations change, aging happens. Sustainability requires adjusting the protocol and movement to fit current circumstances while maintaining the core principles.

- Career change: May require adapting meal preparation and movement timing
- Moving: May require discovering new running routes or gyms
- Aging: May require adjusting exercise intensity while maintaining consistency
- Health changes: May require medical coordination and adjustment

The core principles remain; the specific implementation adapts to circumstances.

Have a Why That Goes Beyond Appearance

Long-term sustainability is strongest when your "why" is deeper than just weight or appearance. Consider:

- Health: Preventing disease, reversing disease, optimizing health
- Longevity: Living long enough to see grandchildren, great-grandchildren
- Capacity: Maintaining ability to do things you love (hiking, sports, travel)
- Identity: "I'm someone who values my health"
- Values: Alignment with values around nature, healing, thriving

A deep "why" sustains motivation through decades, not just months.

COMMON OBSTACLES TO LONG-TERM SUSTAINABILITY AND HOW TO NAVIGATE THEM

Despite best intentions, people often encounter obstacles to long-term adherence. Understanding common obstacles and how to navigate them helps maintain sustainability:

Obstacle 1: "Boredom" with Food

What happens: After months of eating protocol foods, someone feels bored. The foods feel repetitive. The variety seems limited.

Reality: This is often a symptom of not exploring the full range of available foods. There are hundreds of vegetables, legumes, grains, nuts, seeds, and fruits. It's possible to eat protocol foods for a lifetime without repeating the same meal twice.

Navigation:

- Actively explore new foods, such as visit farmer's markets, try cuisines you haven't experienced, experiment with recipes
- Join cooking communities or classes
- Follow plant-based recipe blogs and cookbooks
- Give yourself permission to adventure in your eating

Obstacle 2: Social Pressure and Feeling Different

What happens: People around the individual are eating differently. There's pressure to conform. The individual feels isolated or weird for eating differently.

Reality: This is real and often the single biggest challenge to long-term adherence. It requires navigation.

Navigation:

- Find your community: Others living similarly, whether online or locally
- Don't make it a statement: You don't need to criticize others' choices or be preachy about yours
- Allow flexibility: It's okay to make different choices in social settings sometimes
- Be confident: Your health improvements are real; your choices are valid
- Help others understand: Share your journey; people often become curious and supportive

Obstacle 3: Competing Priorities and Time Constraints

What happens: Life gets busy. Work demands increase. Family situations change. Time for meal preparation and exercise decreases. Adherence becomes harder.

Reality: Life has seasons. Some seasons allow more time for optimal practice; some demand more adaptation. This is normal.

Navigation:

- Simplify when needed: Simple meals can be protocol-aligned; you don't always need complex recipes
- Batch cook efficiently: Having frozen protocol-aligned meals ready for busy weeks
- Adapt exercise: Some movement is always better than no movement; adjust intensity and duration as needed
- Recognize seasons: Busy seasons are temporary; the sustainable foundation remains

Obstacle 4: Feeling "Good Enough" and Letting Adherence Slip

What happens: After months or years of health improvements, someone feels good. They've reached their goals. They gradually relax their adherence. Slowly, adherence decreases and health markers begin worsening.

Reality: This is common. Health is dynamic; maintaining health requires ongoing commitment.

Navigation:

- Understand the permanence: You feel good *because* of the protocol, not in spite of it. Stopping the protocol doesn't maintain the benefits.
- Continue monitoring: Regular health markers keep you aware of your status
- Reconnect with your why: Remind yourself why the protocol matters to you
- Recommit: If adherence has slipped, recommit. It's never too late.

Obstacle 5: Facing Criticism or Judgment

What happens: People criticize the protocol, saying, "It's too extreme," "You're not getting enough protein," "You're obsessed with food," or "You'll get deficiencies." Criticism creates doubt.

Reality: Criticism is common. You're living differently from the majority. This creates friction.

Navigation:

- Understand the science: You know why you're doing this; the evidence supports it.

- Don't need to convince others: You're living for your health, not to convince others.
- Find supportive people: Spend time with people who support your choices.
- Let results speak: Your health improvements are the best argument.
- Ignore unsolicited medical advice: Random people offering health criticism aren't qualified doctors with full knowledge of your situation.

The Long-Term Vision: Decades of Optimal Health

Ultimately, long-term sustainability is about creating a life where optimal health is simply how you live. Not something you're working toward, but something you're living.

A person who has sustained the Energy Restoration Protocol for ten, twenty, thirty or more years:

- Experiences consistent, abundant energy.
- Maintains optimal weight and body composition throughout life.
- Maintains excellent cognitive function; doesn't experience age-related cognitive decline.
- Maintains excellent physical capacity; doesn't experience typical age-related loss of function.
- Avoids the chronic diseases that plague their peers.
- Has exceptional quality of life that is free from disease, free from medications (or minimal medications), and free from fear about health.
- Often becomes an inspiration to those around them, such as family members, friends, and younger people who see this person thriving.

This is not utopian fantasy. This is what becomes possible with decades-long implementation of the protocol combined with consistent, age-appropriate movement.

Moving Forward

Long-term sustainability is not about perfection. It's about consistency. It's about making the protocol your normal way of living. It's about integrating movement into your daily life as naturally as breathing. It's about building a life where health is simply how you live, not something you have to fight for.

The final chapter of this manifesto addresses the philosophical and personal dimension: what it means to take responsibility for your own energy, to acknowledge that your health is ultimately your choice, and to step into personal power around your health.

19

YOUR ENERGY,
YOUR RESPONSIBILITY,
YOUR POWER

Reclaiming Health Through Personal Choice and Alignment with Nature

THE MOMENT OF REALIZATION

There's a moment that comes for many people implementing the Energy Restoration Protocol. It usually happens somewhere around Month 2 or 3, when the health improvements are undeniable.

Maybe it's a woman who hasn't felt this energetic in fifteen years, or a man who's shocked to discover his blood pressure has normalized without medication, or someone who realizes their depression has lifted and they're genuinely happy.

In that moment, something shifts. A realization emerges that often takes the form of a question: "If I can reverse this disease through food and lifestyle changes, that means . . . I could have prevented it in the first place. That means . . . I had more control over my health than I believed."

This realization can feel simultaneously liberating and uncomfortable. Liberating because it means the future is not fixed; you have more power over your health than you thought. Uncomfortable because it means acknowledging that the past circumstances that created disease were, at least partially, within your control.

This chapter addresses this realization. It explores what it means to take personal responsibility for your own energy and health. It explores the empowerment that comes from understanding that you have more power over your health than you've been led to believe. And it explores how this understanding transforms not just your health, but your relationship to life itself.

The Victim Narrative vs. the Empowerment Narrative

We live in a medical and cultural system that has trained us into a particular story about health. Let's call it the victim narrative:

> **The Victim Narrative:** "Health problems are something that happen to you. You're either genetically predisposed (and therefore it's inevitable), or you got unlucky (bad genes, bad environment, bad luck), or you're getting old (and decline is just what happens). Your doctor is responsible for fixing your problems. Medications are the solution. You're a passive recipient of whatever health circumstances arise. You do your best, but ultimately, your health is not really in your control."

This narrative is deeply embedded in our culture. It's in the language we use ("I got diabetes," as if disease is something that happens to you rather than something your body created in response to conditions you've been creating). It's in the medical system (you go to the doctor and receive a diagnosis and medications; you're not an active participant in your healing). It's in the media (disease campaigns focus on risk factors and genetics, implying inevitability).

The victim narrative creates a particular relationship to health: resignation, dependence on medical systems, belief in inevitability.

The Energy Restoration Protocol requires and enables a different narrative. Let's call it the empowerment narrative:

> **The Empowerment Narrative:** "My health is the result of the conditions I create through my daily choices. The foods I eat, the movement I engage in, the stress I manage these create either health or disease. I have far more control over my health than I've been led to believe. Yes, genetics matter. Yes, the environment matters. But my daily choices matter enormously. When disease emerges, it's not something that happened to me; it's information about the conditions I've been creating. I have the power to change those conditions and reverse disease. My doctor is a resource and partner, but my health is ultimately my responsibility."

The empowerment narrative creates a different relationship to health: agency, responsibility, possibility.

THE DIFFERENCE THIS MAKES

This distinction between victim and empowerment narratives is not just semantic. It's foundational to whether someone maintains health changes long term.

Someone operating from the victim narrative might implement the protocol temporarily, see improvements, then stop believing it's necessary (because the improvements feel miraculous, not the result of their choices). Or they might maintain it while blaming external circumstances when struggles arise ("If only I had the time/money/support . . ."). They tend to view the protocol as something they're doing for external reasons (to please a doctor, to look better) rather than for internal reasons (because it's how they want to live).

Someone operating from the empowerment narrative understands that their daily choices create their health. The protocol isn't something they're doing; it's how they're living. When they face obstacles, they problem-solve rather than surrender. When they're tempted to deviate, they consider, "Is this what I want to create in my body?" They maintain the protocol indefinitely because they understand that their health is their responsibility and their creation.

Long-term sustainability lives in the empowerment narrative.

You Have More Power Than You Think

One of the most transformative insights that comes from understanding the Energy Restoration Protocol is realizing the extraordinary power you have over your own health. This power is far greater than most people have been led to believe.

THE EVIDENCE OF YOUR POWER

Look at disease reversal: In Sections 2 and 3 of this manifesto, we saw people reversing cardiovascular disease, Type 2 diabetes, obesity, depression, and anxiety. These aren't genetic inevitabilities being overcome through miraculous medications. These are energy dysfunctions being reversed through changes in daily choices.

If disease can be reversed through daily choices, then disease could have been prevented through different daily choices.

This is radical because it means the diseases that many people accept as inevitable are actually preventable and reversible.

Look at disease prevention: We saw families preventing disease across multiple generations through the Energy Restoration Protocol. Their children never developed the chronic diseases that plague processed-food-consuming populations. Their grandchildren grow up with optimal health as their baseline.

If disease can be prevented, then generations of disease are preventable. The multigenerational disease patterns that seem inevitable are actually created by multigenerational dietary and lifestyle patterns. Change the patterns, and the disease disappears.

Look at aging and physical capacity: We saw a sixty-six-year-old runner maintaining athletic performance that exceeds most forty year olds, with health markers indicating a biological age twenty years younger than chronological age.

If this level of vitality and capacity is possible at sixty-six, then the typical age-related decline is not inevitable. It's the result of the conditions created through diet and lifestyle. Change the conditions, and aging can be dramatically different.

These examples are not exceptional miracles. They're the normal results of addressing energy dysfunction through the Energy Restoration Protocol. They're available to anyone willing to make the changes.

This is your power: the power to create your health through your daily choices.

THE RESPONSIBILITY THAT COMES WITH POWER

Power and responsibility are inseparable. Once you understand that you have power over your health, you also understand that you have responsibility for your health.

This can feel uncomfortable. If you get sick, you can't blame your genes, or your doctor, or your bad luck. You have to ask, "What conditions was I creating through my daily choices that allowed disease to emerge?"

This is not about shame or blame. It's about clarity. Understanding responsibility means understanding causation. It means understanding that you're not a victim of your health; you're the creator of it.

This understanding is actually liberating, not burdensome. Because if you created the conditions that led to disease, you can create different conditions that lead to health. You have the power.

The Power of Choice: You Have More Agency Than You Believe

Many people feel trapped by their circumstances. "I can't afford organic vegetables," "I don't have time to cook," "My family won't support healthy eating," "I work too much to exercise."

These obstacles are real. But they're often more limiting than they need to be. They're frequently masking a deeper belief: "I don't have a choice."

The truth is more nuanced—you may not have unlimited choices, but you always have choices. And the choices you do have matter enormously.

THE POWER OF SMALL CHOICES

Consider the moment at the grocery store when you choose between processed food and whole food. You have a choice. That single choice doesn't seem huge. But multiply it across weeks and months and the choices accumulate. The accumulation of small choices creates your health.

For example, the moment when you choose to take a fifteen-minute walk instead of sitting. A single walk doesn't transform health. But accumulated across weeks and months, the accumulation of movement creates physical capacity and well-being.

Or the moment when you choose to have a conversation with someone instead of staying isolated with your worries. A single conversation doesn't transform mental health. But accumulated across weeks and months, the accumulation of connection creates resilience and joy.

These small choices don't feel heroic or empowering at the moment. But they are. Because they are the accumulation of small choices that creates everything: your health, your capacity, your quality of life.

You have more agency than you realize, and it lives in these small choices.

REMOVING THE ILLUSION OF POWERLESSNESS

Many people operate under the belief that they're powerless over their health. "My genes determine my health," "Aging means decline," "I'm stuck with what I was born with."

These beliefs create a sense of powerlessness. And powerlessness creates resignation.

But these beliefs are not true. What's true is:

- Your genes influence your health, but they don't determine it. The conditions you create matter as much as genetics.
- Aging is a process, but it's not declining. Aging can be vitality and continued optimization if conditions are right.
- You're not stuck with what you were born with. You can fundamentally change your health, your capacity, your life.

Removing the illusion of powerlessness is the first step to stepping into your actual power.

Understanding Energy Dysfunction: How It Changes Your Relationship with Health

Once you understand that all chronic disease stems from energy system dysfunction, your relationship with health fundamentally changes.

Rather than seeing disease as random misfortune or genetic destiny, you see it as information. Disease is your body telling you, "The conditions you're creating are not supporting my energy system. I need something different."

This is profoundly different from the victim narrative, where disease seems like bad luck that happens to you.

DISEASE AS INFORMATION, NOT PUNISHMENT

Consider someone who develops Type 2 diabetes. In the victim narrative, this is bad luck or genetic destiny. "My family has diabetes. I was destined to get it." Resignation follows.

In the energy dysfunction framework, diabetes is information: "Your energy system is dysregulated. Your insulin signaling is broken. Your metabolism is not functioning optimally. The foods you've been eating refined carbohydrates, processed foods are creating this dysfunction. Your body is telling you that it needs something different."

This information is valuable. It's not punishment. It's not destiny. It's your body communicating.

When you understand the communication, you can respond. You can provide what your body is asking for: energy optimization through whole foods, insulin sensitivity restoration through reduced refined carbohydrates, metabolic healing through nutrient abundance.

The disease can then be reversed. Not despite the disease, but by listening to what it's telling you and providing what's needed.

HEALTH AS COMMUNICATION TOO

Just as disease is communication, health is communication. When you feel energetic, sleeping well, cognitively sharp, emotionally stable, your body is communicating, "The conditions I'm in are supporting my energy system. Keep going."

Understanding health as communication helps you maintain it. Rather than taking health for granted, you listen to what your body is telling you about what supports it. You notice certain foods make you feel better, certain movements make you feel better, certain sleep patterns support energy, certain stress management practices support resilience.

You're not following arbitrary rules. You're learning to communicate with your own body about what it needs.

Vision: Creating the Future You Want

Understanding your power and responsibility creates an opportunity: you can intentionally create the future you want, rather than accepting whatever trajectory emerges.

ENVISIONING YOUR BEST HEALTH

Take a moment to envision your health at various points in the future. Not what you fear might happen. Not what's "normal" for aging. But what's actually possible if you create the conditions for optimal health:

In one year: What would be different if all your metabolic markers were optimal? If your energy was abundant? If disease markers had reversed? If you were sleeping well and thinking clearly?

In five years: What would be different if these optimal conditions had been maintained? What capacity would you have? What would you be able to do? How would you feel?

In ten years: If you continued creating conditions for optimal health, how would you age? Would you be stronger or weaker than your peers? Would you have more or less energy? More or less capacity?

In twenty years: Imagine reaching older age in excellent health rather than managing chronic disease. What would be different? What would be possible?

This isn't fantasy. This is what becomes possible through the Energy Restoration Protocol maintained consistently.

CHOOSING YOUR VISION

The question is not: "What will happen to me?" The question is: "What do I want to create?"

Once you understand that you have power over your health, you get to choose. You get to choose the future you want to create.

Do you want to create a future of vitality or decline? Do you want to create a future of abundance or depletion? Do you want to create a future where you're aging backward (getting healthier and stronger as you age) or aging forward (getting weaker and more diseased)?

You get to choose. And the choice you make right now, with your food choices, your movement, your stress management is creating that future.

THE RIPPLE EFFECT: YOUR TRANSFORMATION INFLUENCES OTHERS

When you transform your health through the Energy Restoration Protocol, the transformation doesn't stay contained to you. It ripples outward.

Your family sees your health improvements. They become curious. They ask questions. Some begin implementing the protocol themselves. The health of your family transforms.

Your friends see your energy and vitality. They ask what you're doing differently. You share your journey. Some become interested. They implement the protocol. Their health transforms.

Your workplace sees your improved productivity, focus, and energy. They notice. Colleagues ask. You influence workplace culture around health.

Your community sees examples of health and vitality in people around them. The possibility of health becomes more visible. More people begin asking questions.

This ripple effect is profound because it's not just your health transforming. It's entire systems families, workplaces, communities beginning to shift toward health optimization rather than disease management.

YOUR TRANSFORMATION AS PERMISSION

One of the most powerful aspects of your transformation is that it becomes permission for others. When people see you thrive, live fully, maintain excellent health, they think: "If they can do it, maybe I can too."

Your transformation is proof of possibility. It's proof that disease reversal is achievable. That prevention is possible. That vitality in later years is possible. That the trajectory they thought was inevitable is actually changeable.

By living your best health, you give others permission to pursue theirs.

IN NATURE WE TRUST: A Philosophy of Life

The title of this manifesto "IN NATURE WE TRUST" points to something beyond diet and disease. It points to a philosophy about a way of relating to yourself, your body, nature, and the world.

WHAT DOES IT MEAN TO TRUST NATURE?

For thousands of years and across countless cultures, humans evolved eating foods provided by nature: plants in their whole forms, as nature provided them. Our bodies are optimized for these foods. Our mitochondria function best with these foods. Our brains develop optimally with these foods.

In the last fifty to one hundred years, we've largely abandoned foods as nature provides them and replaced them with processed foods as industry designs them. The result: epidemic levels of chronic disease.

To "trust nature" means recognizing that nature's design millions of years of evolution is far more sophisticated than industry's design (150 years of processed food production). It means returning to what nature provides: whole plant foods that nourished humans for millennia.

This is not sentimentality. This is not romanticism. This is recognizing that nature's design works. It creates health. Industry's design creates disease.

NATURE AS PARTNER, NOT ENEMY

Western medicine has often framed nature as something to be conquered or controlled. Disease is an enemy to be fought. Aging is an enemy to be fought. The body is a machine to be repaired.

IN NATURE WE TRUST frames nature differently—not as an enemy to be conquered, but as a partner to be aligned with.

Your body is not a machine. It's a living, intelligent system evolved over millions of years. It's not your enemy; it's trying to help you. When disease emerges, it's not attacking you; it's communicating that something needs to change.

Nature's solutions are not always what we expect. Sometimes the solution to fatigue is not rest but movement. Sometimes the solution to anxiety is not medication but optimal nutrition. Sometimes the solution to disease is not fighting harder but surrendering to what nature actually needs.

When you align with nature, you stop fighting and start cooperating. You stop trying to control and start listening. You stop trying to fix and start healing.

IN NATURE WE TRUST AS PERSONAL PRACTICE

At its deepest level, IN NATURE WE TRUST is a personal practice. It means:

Trusting your body: Not assuming it's broken or against you, but recognizing its intelligence and cooperating with it.

Trusting nature's foods: Trusting that whole plant foods as nature provides them are exactly what your body needs.

Trusting the process: Understanding that health restoration takes time. That your body has extraordinary capacity for healing if given the right conditions.

Trusting yourself: Recognizing that you have power over your health. That you can make choices that matter. That you can create the health you want.

Trusting life: Recognizing that living in alignment with nature both external nature and your own nature creates not just health, but meaning, purpose, and joy.

THE DAILY PRACTICE: WHERE PHILOSOPHY MEETS ACTION

IN NATURE WE TRUST is not just philosophy. It's a practice. It's the small choices you make daily, repeatedly, across years and decades:

The choice to eat whole plant foods instead of processed foods. That's IN NATURE WE TRUST.

The choice to move your body in ways that feel natural and joyful. That's IN NATURE WE TRUST.

The choice to trust your body's signals and respond to them. That's IN NATURE WE TRUST.

The choice to spend time in nature outside, feeling the earth, breathing fresh air. That's IN NATURE WE TRUST.

The choice to slow down and rest when your body signals that it needs rest. That's IN NATURE WE TRUST.

The choice to prioritize your health even when it means saying no to things that don't serve you. That's IN NATURE WE TRUST.

The choice to take responsibility for your health rather than surrendering it to others. That's IN NATURE WE TRUST.

These daily choices, accumulated across time, create a life. A life of health. A life of vitality. A life of genuine freedom.

The Closing Vision: Health as Freedom

At its essence, this entire manifesto is about freedom. Freedom from disease. Freedom from medications. Freedom from fear about your health. Freedom from the belief that you're powerless.

Imagine a world where:

- Children grow up with optimal health as their baseline. They never develop the chronic diseases that plague their grandparents' generation.
- Young adults maintain energy and capacity because they understand how to nourish their bodies.
- Middle-aged adults don't experience the health decline that's currently "normal" for their age.
- Elderly people maintain cognitive sharpness, physical capacity, and independence rather than experiencing typical decline.
- Disease is rare rather than common. Health is the baseline.
- People are free from medications and medical appointments dominated by chronic disease management.
- Health care systems shift from disease management to prevention and support of optimal health.
- People have energy and capacity for meaningful work, deep relationships, and engaged living.

This is not fantasy. This is what becomes possible when populations embrace the Energy Restoration Protocol and the IN NATURE WE TRUST philosophy.

This is the future available to you, your family, your community. Not someday. Not maybe. But available now, through the choices you make starting today.

Your Choice

This manifesto has given you information. You now understand:

- That all chronic disease stems from energy system dysfunction.
- That energy system dysfunction can be prevented and reversed through the Energy Restoration Protocol.
- That disease prevention is superior to disease management.
- That you have far more power over your health than you've been led to believe.
- That this power comes with responsibility.
- That your transformation influences others.
- That health is freedom.

The question now is: What will you do with this information?
You can:

- Share it with others. Your transformation becomes their permission.
- Implement it for yourself. Your health becomes your anchor, your foundation, your freedom.
- Integrate it into your family. Multigenerational health transformation begins.
- Use it to influence your community. Health becomes visible. Possibility becomes real.

Or you can close this book and return to your previous patterns, knowing what you know, and accept the trajectory that follows.

The choice is yours. And the choice matters. It will determine not just your health, but your quality of life, your capacity, your vitality, your freedom.

Final Words: IN NATURE WE TRUST

Life is Energy and Energy is Life.

You are not broken. Your body is not your enemy. Disease is not your destiny.

You have power. More power than you realize. The power to restore your health. The power to prevent disease. The power to create vitality. The power to influence others.

Use your power. Make the choices. Trust nature. Trust your body. Trust yourself.

IN NATURE WE TRUST. In your own nature we trust. In your power, your choice, your responsibility, your freedom, we trust.

Your health is not something that happens to you. It's something you create. Create wisely. Choose well. Live fully.

EPILOGUE:
The Beginning

This manifesto has explored energy restoration in detail. From the foundational philosophy that all disease stems from energy dysfunction, through the practical protocol for energy restoration, through disease reversal case studies, through the integration of protocol into real life across diverse circumstances, to the long-term sustainability that allows decades of optimal health.

But this manifesto is not the end. It's the beginning.

The real work, the real transformation happens in your life. In the kitchen where you prepare meals. In the moments when you choose movement. In the conversations where you share your journey. In the years and decades where you live the protocol and experience its benefits.

This manifesto provides the framework. But you provide the implementation. You provide the commitment. You provide the daily choices that accumulate into a life of health.

The Energy Restoration Protocol works. Science is sound. The evidence is overwhelming. Hundreds of thousands of people have experienced transformation through this protocol.

You can too.

Your best health is available to you. Not someday. Not when circumstances are perfect. But right now, through the choices you make today.

IN NATURE WE TRUST.

Life is Energy and Energy is Life.

ACKNOWLEDGMENTS

This book represents over sixteen years of commitment to a Raw Food lifestyle, and I am deeply grateful to those who supported this journey and helped bring this manifesto to life.

To my mother, whose birthday celebration on December 6, 2009, marked the beginning of this extraordinary journey.

To Dr. Shrenik Shah, MD, whose medical expertise and decades of experience on health transformation with Plant Based Raw food provided the scientific validation at the heart of this work.

To my family, Manisha, Jesal, Shivam, Dwip, Simit, Rajshi, Isha,
Sonia, Carolina, whose support helped shape this project.

To the Raw Foodiest Family, my clients and community, whose transformations continue to inspire and validate this path.

And to Nature itself, the ultimate teacher and healer.

IN NATURE WE TRUST.

NOTES

Chapter 1

1 Atkinson, D.E., et al. (2008). "ATP: Its Use in Cells," in Molecular Biology of the Cell, 5th ed. Garland Science; also van Holde, K.E., Mathews, C.R., & Ahern, K.G. (1998). Biochemistry, 3rd ed. Pearson Education.

2 Berg, J.M., Tymoczko, J.L., & Stryer, L. (2012). *Biochemistry*, 7th ed. W.H. Freeman and Company; also Campbell, N.A., Reece, J.B., & Meacham, C.A. (2015). *Campbell Biology*, 11th ed. Pearson Education. Chapter on Cellular Respiration and ATP Production.

3 Wallace, D.C. (2012). "Mitochondria and Cancer." *Nature Reviews Cancer*, *12*(10), 685–698; also Nunnari, J., & Suomalainen, A. (2012). "Mitochondria: In Sickness and in Health." *Cell*, *148*(6), 1145–1159.

4 Raichle, M.E., & Gusnard, D.A. (2002). "Appraising the Brain's Energy Budget." Proceedings of the National Academy of Sciences, *99*(16), 10237–10239; also Kety, S.S. (1957). "The Physiology of the Cerebral Circulation." Journal of Cerebral Blood Flow & Metabolism, *16*(1), 4–17.

5 Ashcroft, F.M., & Rorsman, P. (2012). "Diabetes Mellitus and the β-cell: the Last Ten Years." Cell, *148*(6), 1160–1171; also Henquin, J.C. (2000). "Triggering and Amplification of Insulin Secretion by Glucose in β-cells." *American Journal of Physiology*, *279*(4), E540-E557.

6 Prentki, M., & Nolan, C.J. (2006). "Islet Beta Cell Failure in Type 2 Diabetes." *The Journal of Clinical Investigation*, *116*(7), 1802–1812; also DeFronzo, R.A. (2009). "From the Triumvirate to the Ominous Octet: A New Paradigm for the Treatment of Type 2 Diabetes Mellitus." *Diabetes*, *58*(4), 773–795. Beta cell dysfunction and progressive insulin secretion failure mechanisms in Type 2 Diabetes from cellular and clinical studies.

7 Lustig, R.H. (2013). *Fat Chance: Beating the Odds Against Sugar, Processed Food, Obesity, and Disease*. Hudson Street Press; also Ludwig, D.S. (2002). "The Glycemic Index: Physiological Mechanisms Relating to Obesity, Diabetes, and Cardiovascular Disease." *Journal of the American College of Nutrition*, *21*(2), 146–151. Glucose spikes, insulin response, and de novo lipogenesis mechanisms from metabolic biochemistry and nutritional science.

8 Manach, C., et al. (2004). "Polyphenols: Food Sources and Bioavailability." *American Journal of Clinical Nutrition*, *79*(5), 727–747; also Scalbert, A., et al. (2005). "Dietary Polyphenols and the Prevention of Diseases." *Critical Reviews in Food Science and Nutrition*, *45*(4), 287–306.

Chapter 2

1 Taubes, G. (2016). *The Case Against Sugar*. Knopf Publishing; also Moss, M. (2013). *Salt, Sugar, Fat: How the Food Giants Hooked Us*. Random House. Historical sugar consumption data from U.S. Department of Agriculture and USDA Economic Research Service archives.

2 Teicholz, N. (2014). *The Big Fat Surprise: Why Butter, Meat and Cheese Belong in a Healthy Diet*. Simon & Schuster; also Taubes, G. (2007). *Good Calories, Bad Calories: Challenging the Big-Fat Consensus Theory of Diet, Disease, and Health*. Knopf Publishing. Historical analysis of McGovern Committee dietary goals (1977) and sugar industry influence documented in Senate records and industry archives.

3 Astrup, A., et al. (2011). "The Role of Reducing Intakes of Saturated Fat in the Prevention of Cardiovascular Disease: Where Does the Evidence Stand in 2010?" *American Journal of Clinical Nutrition*, 93(4), 684–688; also Ludwig, D.S., & Willett, W.C. (2013). "The High-Fat Diet Question." *JAMA*, 310(1), 33–34. Analysis of low-fat diet effects on satiety and carbohydrate consumption patterns from multiple observational and intervention studies.

4 Monteiro, C.A., et al. (2018). "Ultra-processed Foods: What They Are and How to Identify Them." *Public Health Nutrition*, 19(1), 1–6; also Moss, M. (2013). *Salt, Sugar, Fat: How the Food Giants Hooked Us*. Random House. Study cited from U.S. Department of Agriculture Nutrient Database Analysis.

5 American Heart Association. (2020). *Heart Disease and Stroke Statistics—2020 Update*. American Heart Association; also Marmot, M.G., & McDowall, M.E. (1986). "Mortality Decline and Widening Social Inequalities." *The Lancet*, 2(8501), 274–276. Historical data on coronary heart disease mortality trends from CDC and World Health Organization databases.

6 Mozaffarian, D., et al. (2015). "Trans Fats and Cardiovascular Disease." *New England Journal of Medicine*, 354(15), 1601–1613; also Keys, A. (1970). "Coronary Heart Disease in Seven Countries." *Circulation*, 41(4 Supplement 1), I-1 to I-211. Historical epidemiological data on heart disease mortality from CDC and American Heart Association archives (1920–1950).

7 Willett, W.C. (2002). "Diet and Cancer: One View at the Start of the Millennium." *Cancer Epidemiology, Biomarkers & Prevention*, 10(1), 3–8; also Doll, R., & Peto, R. (1981). "The Causes of Cancer: Quantitative Estimates of Avoidable Risks of Cancer in the United States Today." *Journal of the National Cancer Institute*, 66(6), 1191–1308. Cancer incidence data from National Cancer Institute Surveillance, Epidemiology, and End Results (SEER) program, 1950–2020.

8 Centers for Disease Control and Prevention. (2020). *National Diabetes Statistics Report*. CDC; also Saeedi, P., et al. (2019). "Global and Regional Diabetes Prevalence Estimates for 2019 and Projections by 2030." *Diabetes Research and Clinical Practice*, 157, 107843.

9 Willcox, D.C., et al. (2008). "The Okinawan Diet: Health Implications of a Low-Calorie, Nutrient-Dense, Antioxidant-Rich Dietary Pattern Low in Glycemic Load." *Journal of the American College of Nutrition*, 23(5), 369–382; also Wilcox, B.J., Willcox, D.C., & Suzuki, M. (2002). *The Okinawa Program*. Clarkson Potter Publishers.

10 Knowler, W.C., et al. (2002). "Reduction in the Incidence of Type 2 Diabetes with Lifestyle Intervention or Metformin." *The New England Journal of Medicine*, 346(6), 393–403; also Nelson, R.G., et al. (1990). "Epidemiology of Diabetes and Its Vascular Lesions." *Diabetes Care*, 13(Supplement 2), 1–154. Pima Indian diabetes prevalence data from National Institutes of Health Indian Health Service.

11 Kearns, C.E., et al. (2016). "Sugar Industry and Coronary Heart Disease Research: A Historical Analysis of Internal Industry Documents." *JAMA Internal Medicine*, 176(11), 1680–1685; also Taubes, G. (2016). *The Case Against Sugar*. Knopf Publishing. Original

sugar industry documents available through University of California San Francisco Legacy Tobacco Documents Library.

12 Barnard, N.D., et al. (2009). "A Low-Fat Vegan Diet Improves Glycemic Control and Cardiovascular Risk Factors in a Randomized Clinical Trial in Individuals With Type 2 Diabetes." *Diabetes Care, 32*(8), 1433–1438; also Ornish, D., et al. (1998). "Intensive Lifestyle Changes for Reversal of Coronary Heart Disease." *JAMA, 280*(23), 2001–2007. Case reports and clinical outcomes from plant-based nutrition intervention trials demonstrating disease reversal.

Chapter 4

1 Vaya, J., & Mahmood, U. (2006). "Flavonoid Content in Leaf Extracts of the Carob Tree, Ceratonia siliqua (L.), Myrtle, Myrtus communis (L.), and Pistachio, Pistacia lentiscus (L.)." *Journal of Agricultural and Food Chemistry, 54*(20), 7651–7654; also Brand-Miller, J., et al. (2003). "Glycemic Index and Obesity." *American Journal of Clinical Nutrition, 76*(1), 281S-285S. Continuous glucose monitoring studies demonstrating fiber effects on glucose kinetics and glycemic responses.

2 Freedman, M.R., et al. (2008). "The Glycemic Index: Physiological Mechanisms Relating to Obesity, Diabetes, and Cardiovascular Disease." *Journal of the American College of Nutrition, 21*(2), 146–151; also Molnar, D., et al. (2010). "Reality of Continuous Glucose Monitoring Systems (CGMS) in Clinical Practice." *Pediatric Diabetes, 11*(8), 570–577. Continuous glucose monitoring studies comparing whole food vs. processed food glycemic responses from diabetes technology and nutrition research."

Chapter 6

1 O'Keefe, S.J.D., et al. (2015). "Fat, Fibre and Colorectal Cancer Risk in African Americans and Rural Africans." *Nature Communications, 6,* 6342; also Cordain, L., et al. (2005). "Origins and Evolution of the Western Diet: Health Implications for the 21st Century." *American Journal of Clinical Nutrition, 81*(2), 341–354. Bioaccumulation of inflammatory markers and xenobiotics in animal tissue; dietary pattern effects on inflammatory biomarkers from nutritional epidemiology.

2 Vessby, B., et al. (2001). "Substituting Dietary Saturated for Monounsaturated Fat Impairs Insulin Sensitivity in Healthy Men and Women: The KANWU Study." *Diabetologia, 44*(3), 312–319; also Summers, L.K., et al. (2002). "Acute Exposure to Dietary Saturated and trans-Unsaturated Fats Increases Insulin Resistance in Overweight Men." *Metabolism, 51*(8), 972–976.

3 Davignon, J., & Ganz, P. (2004). "Role of Endothelial Dysfunction in Atherosclerosis." *Circulation, 109*(23 Supplement 1), III-27 to III-32; also Vita, J.A., & Keaney, J.F. (2002). "Endothelial Function: A Barometer for Cardiovascular Health." *Circulation, 106*(6), 640–642. Mechanism studies on LDL cholesterol and saturated fat effects on vascular endothelium from NIH and American Heart Association research.

4 Riccardi, G., et al. (2008). "Dietary Fiber and Indicators of Insulin Resistance." *Nutrients, 1*(1), 23–33; also Jenkins, D.J., et al. (2008). "Glycemic Index: Overview of Implications for Health and Disease." *American Journal of Clinical Nutrition, 76*(1), 266S-273S.

Phytochemical and fiber effects on glucose metabolism from multiple meta-analyses and clinical intervention studies.

Chapter 14

1   Yau, J.W., et al. (2012). "Global Prevalence and Major Risk Factors of Diabetic Retinopathy." *Diabetes Care*, *35*(3), 556–564; also Kempen, J.H., et al. (2004). "The Prevalence of Diabetic Retinopathy Among Adults in the United States." *Archives of Ophthalmology*, *122*(4), 552–563.

2   Tesfaye, S., et al. (2010). "Diabetic Neuropathies: Update on Definitions, Diagnostic Criteria, Estimation of Severity, and Treatments." *Diabetes Care*, *33*(12), 2285–2293; also Callaghan, B.C., et al. (2012). "Prevalence of Diabetic Neuropathy and Relation to Glycemic Control and Potential Risk Factors." *Diabetes Care*, *35*(8), 1746–1748.

3   Gross, J.L., et al. (2005). "Diabetic Nephropathy: Diagnosis, Prevention, and Treatment." *Diabetes Care*, *28*(1), 164–176; also Molitch, M.E., et al. (2004). "Nephropathy in Diabetes." *Diabetes Care*, *27*(Supplement 1), S79-S83.

BIBLIOGRAPHY

American Heart Association. (2020). Heart Disease and Stroke Statistics—2020 Update. American Heart Association.

Ashcroft, F.M., & Rorsman, P. (2012). Diabetes mellitus and the β-cell: The last ten years. *Cell*, *148*(6), 1160–1171.

Astrup, A., et al. (2011). The role of reducing intakes of saturated fat in the prevention of cardiovascular disease: Where does the evidence stand in 2010? *American Journal of Clinical Nutrition*, *93*(4), 684–688.

Atkinson, D.E., et al. (2007). ATP: Its use in cells. In *Molecular biology of the cell* (5th ed.). Garland Science.

Barnard, N.D., et al. (2009). A low-fat vegan diet improves glycemic control and cardiovascular risk factors in a randomized clinical trial in individuals with type 2 diabetes. *Diabetes Care*, *32*(8), 1433–1438.

Berg, J.M., Tymoczko, J.L., & Stryer, L. (2012). *Biochemistry* (7th ed.). W.H. Freeman and Company.

Brand-Miller, J., et al. (2003). Glycemic index and obesity. *American Journal of Clinical Nutrition*, *76*(1), 281S-285S.

Callaghan, B.C., et al. (2012). Prevalence of diabetic neuropathy and relation to glycemic control and potential risk factors. *Diabetes Care*, *35*(8), 1746–1748.

Campbell, N.A., Reece, J.B., & Meacham, C.A. (2015). *Campbell biology* (11th ed.). Pearson Education.

Centers for Disease Control and Prevention. (2020). National Diabetes Statistics Report. CDC.

Cordain, L., et al. (2005). Origins and evolution of the Western diet: Health implications for the 21st Century. *American Journal of Clinical Nutrition*, *81*(2), 341–354.

Craft, S., et al. (2009). Intranasal insulin effects on cognition and Alzheimer's disease biomarkers in mild cognitive impairment. *Journal of Alzheimer's Disease*, *15*(2), 301–310.

Davignon, J., & Ganz, P. (2004). Role of endothelial dysfunction in atherosclerosis. *Circulation*, *109*(23 Supplement 1), III-27 to III-32.

DeFronzo, R.A. (2009). From the triumvirate to the ominous octet: A new paradigm for the treatment of type 2 diabetes mellitus. *Diabetes*, *58*(4), 773–795.

Doll, R., & Peto, R. (1981). The causes of cancer: Quantitative estimates of avoidable risks of cancer in the United States today. *Journal of the National Cancer Institute*, *66*(6), 1191–1308.

Freedman, M.R., et al. (2008). The glycemic index: Physiological mechanisms relating to obesity, diabetes, and cardiovascular disease. *Journal of the American College of Nutrition*, *21*(2), 146–151.

Gross, J.L., et al. (2005). Diabetic nephropathy: Diagnosis, prevention, and treatment. *Diabetes Care*, *28*(1), 164–176.

Henquin, J.C. (2000). Triggering and amplification of insulin secretion by glucose in β-cells. *American Journal of Physiology*, *279*(4), E540-E557.

Jenkins, D.J., et al. (2008). Glycemic index: Overview of implications for health and disease. *American Journal of Clinical Nutrition, 76*(1), 266S-273S.

Kearns, C.E., et al. (2016). Sugar industry and coronary heart disease research: A historical analysis of internal industry documents. *JAMA Internal Medicine, 176*(11), 1680–1685.

Kempen, J.H., et al. (2004). The prevalence of diabetic retinopathy among adults in the United States. *Archives of Ophthalmology, 122*(4), 552–563.

Kety, S.S. (1957). The physiology of the cerebral circulation. *Journal of Cerebral Blood Flow & Metabolism, 16*(1), 4–17.

Keys, A. (1970). Coronary heart disease in seven countries. *Circulation, 41*(4 Supplement 1), I-1 to I-211.

Knowler, W.C., et al. (2002). Reduction in the incidence of type 2 diabetes with lifestyle intervention or metformin. *The New England Journal of Medicine, 346*(6), 393–403.

Ludwig, D.S. (2002). The glycemic index: Physiological mechanisms relating to obesity, diabetes, and cardiovascular disease. *Journal of the American College of Nutrition, 21*(2), 146–151.

Ludwig, D.S., & Willett, W.C. (2013). The high-fat diet question. *JAMA, 310*(1), 33–34.

Lustig, R.H. (2013). *Fat chance: Beating the odds against sugar, processed food, obesity, and disease.* Hudson Street Press.

Manach, C., et al. (2004). Polyphenols: food sources and bioavailability. *American Journal of Clinical Nutrition, 79*(5), 727–747.

Marmot, M.G., & McDowall, M.E. (1986). Mortality decline and widening social inequalities. *The Lancet, 2*(8501), 274–276.

McGill, C.R., et al. (2013). Role of vinegar in metabolic health and glucose control. *Nutrition Reviews, 73*(3), 175–183.

Molitch, M.E., et al. (2004). Nephropathy in diabetes. *Diabetes Care, 27*(Supplement 1), S79-S83.

Molnar, D., et al. (2010). Reality of continuous glucose monitoring systems (CGMS) in clinical practice. *Pediatric Diabetes, 11*(8), 570–577.

Monteiro, C.A., et al. (2018). Ultra-processed foods: What they are and how to identify them. *Public Health Nutrition, 19*(1), 1–6.

Moss, M. (2013). *Salt, sugar, fat: How the food giants hooked us.* Random House.

Mozaffarian, D., et al. (2015). Trans fats and cardiovascular disease. *New England Journal of Medicine, 354*(15), 1601–1613.

Nelson, R.G., et al. (1990). Epidemiology of diabetes and its vascular lesions. *Diabetes Care, 13*(Supplement 2), 1–154.

Nunnari, J. & Suomalainen, A. (2012). Mitochondria: In sickness and in health. *Cell, 148*(6), 1145–1159.

O'Keefe, S.J.D., et al. (2015). Fat, fiber and colorectal cancer risk in African Americans and rural Africans. *Nature Communications, 6,* 6342.

Ornish, D., et al. (1998). Intensive lifestyle changes for reversal of coronary heart disease. *JAMA, 280*(23), 2001–2007.

Prentki, M., & Nolan, C.J. (2006). Islet beta cell failure in type 2 diabetes. *The Journal of Clinical Investigation, 116*(7), 1802–1812.

Raichle, M.E. & Gusnard, D.A. (2002). Appraising the brain's energy budget. *Proceedings of the National Academy of Sciences, 99*(16), 10237–10239.

Riccardi, G., et al. (2008). Dietary fiber and indicators of insulin resistance. *Nutrients, 1*(1), 23–33.

Saeedi, P., et al. (2019). Global and regional diabetes prevalence estimates for 2019 and projections by 2030. *Diabetes Research and Clinical Practice, 157*, 107843.

Scalbert, A., et al. (2005). Dietary polyphenols and the prevention of diseases. *Critical Reviews in Food Science and Nutrition, 45*(4), 287–306.

Summers, L.K., et al. (2002). Acute exposure to dietary saturated and trans-unsaturated fats increases insulin resistance in overweight men. *Metabolism, 51*(8), 972–976.

Taubes, G. (2007). *Good calories, bad calories: Challenging the big-fat consensus theory of diet, disease, and health*. Knopf Publishing.

Taubes, G. (2016). *The case against sugar*. Knopf Publishing.

Teicholz, N. (2014). *The big fat surprise: Why butter, meat and cheese belong in a healthy diet*. Simon and Schuster.

Tesfaye, S., et al. (2010). Diabetic neuropathies: Update on definitions, diagnostic criteria, estimation of severity, and treatments. *Diabetes Care, 33*(12), 2285–2293.

Tipton, K.F. (2014). The enzymes of detoxication. *Current Topics in Medicinal Chemistry, 13*(12), 1371–1390.

van Holde, K.E., Mathews, C.R., & Ahern, K.G. (1998). *Biochemistry* (3rd ed.). Pearson Education.

Vessby, B., et al. (2001). Substituting dietary saturated for monounsaturated fat impairs insulin sensitivity in healthy men and women: The KANWU study. *Diabetologia, 44*(3), 312–319.

Vita, J.A., & Keaney, J.F. (2002). Endothelial function: A barometer for cardiovascular health. *Circulation, 106*(6), 640–642.

Wallace, D.C. (2012). Mitochondria and cancer. *Nature Reviews Cancer, 12*(10), 685–698.

Wilcox, B.J., Willcox, D.C., & Suzuki, M. (2002). *The Okinawa program*. Clarkson Potter Publishers.

Willcox, D.C., et al. (2008). The Okinawan diet: Health implications of a low-calorie, nutrient-dense, antioxidant-rich dietary pattern low in glycemic load. *Journal of the American College of Nutrition, 23*(5), 369–382.

Willett, W.C. (2002). Diet and cancer: One view at the start of the millennium. *Cancer Epidemiology, Biomarkers & Prevention, 10*(1), 3–8.

Yau, J.W., et al. (2012). Global prevalence and major risk factors of diabetic retinopathy. *Diabetes Care, 35*(3), 556–564.

GLOSSARY

ACCEPTANCE The ability to embrace change without resistance. In your transformation, acceptance means welcoming the new energy your body experiences as you shift to plant-based raw food. Acceptance removes the struggle and opens the door to lasting change.

BETA CELLS Specialized cells in your pancreas that produce insulin. When you feed them processed foods, they become exhausted and stop working properly. Feed them plant-based raw food, and they regenerate and function optimally again.

BIOLOGICAL ENERGY The measurable energy your cells produce from food. Raw plants activate this energy production. Processed foods deplete it. Your energy level each day directly reflects how efficiently your cells are producing this biological energy.

CELLULAR ENERGY The process by which your cells convert food into usable energy. Think of it like a battery. Raw, plant-based food charges your battery fully. Processed food only partially charges it. The difference is how you feel.

CELLULAR REGENERATION Your body's natural ability to repair and rebuild itself at the cellular level. This happens when you provide it with Mother Nature's foods. Your skin clears. Your energy increases. Your mind sharpens. Your body is rebuilding itself.

COUNTERFEIT FREEDOM The false sense of control you get from eating whatever you want. It feels free in the moment, but it enslaves your body to addiction, lethargy, and poor health. True freedom is controlling what goes into your body.

DAIRY One of the Five Slow Poisons. Animal milk and milk products (cheese, yogurt, butter) are designed by nature for baby animals, not adult humans. They create inflammation, disrupt digestion, and age your body. Eliminate them.

DIABETES PREVENTION PROGRAM (DPP) A landmark clinical study that proved 58 percent reduction in diabetes risk through lifestyle intervention (diet + exercise). This isn't theory - this is science. Your transformation is based on what this study proved is possible.

EMBRACE Week 1 of your thirty-day transformation. You are building mental readiness and comfort with change. Your goal is 40–50 percent plant-based raw food. This week is about acceptance, awareness, and preparing your mind for the power ahead.

EMPOWER Week 2 of your thirty-day transformation. You take action. You eliminate the Five Slow Poisons. You increase discipline. You listen to your body. Your power grows. Your control increases.

ENERGY The fundamental life force that flows through all living things. Your energy level on any given day reflects how efficiently your cells are converting food into fuel. Plant-based raw food maximizes this energy. Processed food destroys it.

FOOD FREEDOM The ability to eat what serves your body, not what enslaves it. True food freedom is choosing foods that make you feel alive, clear, and powerful. It's the ultimate expression of control over your own destiny.

GRAINS One of the Five Slow Poisons. Modern processed grains (wheat, rice, oats, corn) are heavily refined, depleted of nutrition, and spiked with additives. They cause inflammation, digestive issues, and energy crashes. Choose raw vegetables and fruits instead.

GLUCOSE (Blood Sugar) The sugar in your blood that provides energy to your cells. When you eat processed foods and refined sugar, your glucose spikes and crashes. When you eat raw plant-based foods, glucose stays stable, and your energy stays consistent.

HEALTH MANIFESTATION The physical reality of your daily choices. Your skin, energy, weight, mood, and mental clarity are direct reflections of what you eat. Change your food, change your manifestation. Your body is honest—it shows the truth.

HONESTY WITH YOURSELF The most powerful principle in this manifesto. Without it, nothing changes. With it, everything is possible. Being honest means acknowledging what you eat, how you feel, and what you need. Honesty is supreme.

INFLAMMATION Your body's reaction to foods it cannot process efficiently. Processed foods, dairy, grains, and refined sugars cause chronic inflammation. This inflammation ages your body, clouds your mind, and drains your energy. Eliminate the source, reduce inflammation.

IN NATURE WE TRUST™ The core philosophy. When we trust nature's foods (plants made by Mother Nature) over corporate substitutes, we reclaim our health, our energy, and our freedom. This is both scientifically sound and spiritually powerful.

INSULIN RESISTANCE When your cells stop responding to insulin because they've been overwhelmed by processed foods and refined sugar. This is how diabetes develops. The Diabetes Prevention Program proved that lifestyle changes can reverse this before it becomes permanent.

LIFE IS ENERGY and ENERGY IS LIFE The twin philosophy of this manifesto. Everything in nature runs on energy. Your body runs on energy. The question is: What kind of energy are you feeding yourself? Plant-based raw food = pure, alive energy.

LIFESTYLE INTERVENTION The scientific term for changing your diet and exercise habits. This is not medication. This is not surgery. This is you taking control through daily choices. The research proves this works—better than drugs for many conditions.

METABOLIC HEALTH The efficiency with which your body processes food into energy and maintains balance. When you eat plant-based raw food, your metabolism optimizes. Your body becomes an efficient energy machine instead of a struggling, sluggish one.

MITOCHONDRIA The powerhouse of your cells. These tiny organelles convert food into usable energy. They are literally the energy factories of your body. Raw, plant-based food activates them. Processed food exhausts them. Feed your mitochondria right, and you feel alive.

MOTHER NATURE The source of all real food. Foods made by Mother Nature (fruits, vegetables, nuts, seeds, legumes) are perfectly designed to nourish your body. Foods made in factories are designed to profit corporations. Choose Mother Nature.

PLANT-BASED RAW FOOD Food from plants (vegetables, fruits, nuts, seeds, legumes, sprouts) consumed in their natural, uncooked state. This is the foundation of this manifesto. Raw means alive, unaltered, full of enzymes and nutrition.

PROCESSED OILS One of the Five Slow Poisons. Oils extracted from seeds using high heat and chemicals (vegetable, canola, soy oils) are oxidized and toxic to your body. They cause inflammation and damage cellular health. Use whole food sources of fat instead.

REFINED SALT One of the Five Slow Poisons. Table salt has been stripped of minerals and filled with additives. Your body cannot process it efficiently. It contributes to high blood pressure and water retention.

REFINED SUGAR One of the Five Slow Poisons. White sugar, brown sugar, and high-fructose corn syrup are highly processed and addictive. They create energy crashes, feed harmful bacteria in your gut, and age your body. Eliminate them completely.

TRANSCEND Week 4 of your thirty-day transformation. You have transformed. Now you transcend—you move beyond your own transformation to share your wisdom with others. You become a guide. You help others see what's possible.

TRANSFORM Week 3 of your thirty-day transformation. Your body is visibly changing. Your energy is soaring. You are moving your body through.

COMPREHENSIVE DISCLAIMER AND IMPORTANT INFORMATION

Read This Before Implementation

This comprehensive disclaimer provides detailed guidance for implementing the Energy Restoration Protocol safely and effectively.

WHAT THIS MANIFESTO IS (AND ISN'T)

What this manifesto *is*:

- A detailed framework for understanding energy system dysfunction as the root of chronic disease
- The author's personal twenty-one years of documented health transformation and medical data
- Real-world case studies of individuals who have implemented the Energy Restoration Protocol
- Educational content about nutrition, metabolism, and disease prevention
- Practical guidance for dietary and lifestyle changes based on personal experience
- A resource to discuss with your health care provider

What this manifesto *is not*:

- Medical advice or medical diagnosis
- A substitute for professional medical care or consultation
- A clinical trial or peer-reviewed research study
- A guarantee of specific health outcomes for any individual
- An alternative to necessary medical treatment
- A replacement for prescription medications without medical supervision
- A one-size-fits-all solution for all people in all circumstances

IMPORTANT MEDICAL NOTICE

The author is not a licensed physician, registered dietitian, psychologist, or medical professional. This manifesto is based on personal experience and real-world case studies, not clinical trials or peer-reviewed research.

Before implementing significant dietary or lifestyle changes, consult with a quali-fied health care provider. This is especially important if you have:

- Existing chronic health conditions
- Current medications or supplements
- Pregnancy or breastfeeding
- Mental health conditions or psychiatric medications
- Severe or life-threatening conditions
- Autoimmune diseases
- Kidney, liver, or gastrointestinal conditions
- Food allergies or severe intolerances
- Eating disorder history
- Any concerns about your ability to safely implement these changes

SPECIAL POPULATIONS: IMPORTANT CONSIDERATIONS

Pregnancy and Breastfeeding

Do not implement the Energy Restoration Protocol during pregnancy or breastfeeding without explicit permission and guidance from your OB/GYN or midwife.

While Chapter 17 provides guidance for pregnant and breastfeeding women on the protocol, this guidance is for women already established on the protocol or implementing it under professional supervision. The nutritional demands of pregnancy and breastfeeding are extraordinarily high and require careful medical oversight.

Specific concerns requiring medical supervision:

- Adequate caloric intake for fetal development
- Adequate protein for maternal and fetal health
- Adequate B12 (critical for fetal neural development)
- Adequate iron (critical for expanded blood volume and fetal development)
- Adequate DHA (critical for fetal brain development)
- Adequate calcium (critical for fetal bone development)
- Monitoring for gestational diabetes
- Monitoring for preeclampsia

Consult your obstetric provider before making any dietary changes during pregnancy or breastfeeding.

Mental Health Conditions and Psychiatric Medications

Do not discontinue psychiatric medications without explicit medical supervision.

While Chapter 17 describes mental health improvement and medication reduction through the protocol, these changes occurred under psychiatric supervision with careful monitoring. Psychiatric medications serve critical functions in mental health stability and should never be stopped abruptly.

Important guidelines:

- Continue all psychiatric medications as prescribed.
- Inform your psychiatrist or mental health provider about implementing the protocol.
- Work with your provider on any medication adjustments.
- Medication reduction should occur gradually under professional supervision.
- Never stop medications based on reading this manifesto.
- Some psychiatric conditions may require ongoing medication management.
- The protocol supports psychiatric treatment but does not replace it.

If you have severe mental illness, work with your mental health provider before implementing significant dietary changes.

Chronic Kidney Disease or Kidney Complications

Special medical supervision required.

While Chapter 17 addresses diabetes-related kidney disease, people with kidney disease should not implement this protocol without explicit medical supervision. Kidney disease may require specific protein intake management, mineral restrictions, or other considerations.

Important guidelines:

- Work with your nephrologist before implementing dietary changes.
- Kidney function should be monitored during transition.
- Protein intake may need medical guidance.
- Mineral intake (potassium, phosphorus, sodium) may need monitoring.
- Medications may need adjustment as kidney function changes.

Consult your nephrologist before implementing this protocol if you have any kidney disease or kidney complications.

Autoimmune Conditions

Medical supervision recommended.

While the anti-inflammatory effects of the protocol may benefit autoimmune conditions, some individuals with autoimmune disease experience temporary symptom flare-ups during dietary transitions. Additionally, some autoimmune conditions may have specific nutritional considerations.

Important guidelines:

- Work with your rheumatologist or autoimmune disease specialist.
- Monitor for symptom changes carefully.
- Transition gradually rather than abruptly.
- Medications may need adjustment.
- Some autoimmune conditions may require modified protein or specific nutrients.

Consult your autoimmune disease specialist before implementing this protocol.

Severe Chronic Conditions

Medical supervision and careful transition required.

People with severe chronic conditions (advanced diabetes, advanced cardiovascular disease, advanced cancer, advanced neurological conditions, and so on) should not implement the protocol without explicit medical supervision. These conditions often require careful medication management, and dietary changes may affect treatment efficacy.

Consult your health care team if you have severe chronic conditions before implementing this protocol.

MEDICATIONS AND MEDICAL MANAGEMENT

Critical: Medication Changes Require Medical Supervision

Do not make any changes to your medications without consulting your health care provider.

As your health markers improve through the Energy Restoration Protocol, your medications may need adjustment. This requires active medical oversight:

- Blood pressure medications may need reduction or discontinuation.
- Diabetes medications may need adjustment.
- Psychiatric medications may need modification.
- Other medications may need dose changes.
- New medication interactions may emerge.

Work closely with your health care provider on all medication management. Monitor your health markers (blood pressure, blood glucose, and so on) and inform your provider of changes. Your provider can determine if medication adjustments are appropriate.

Medication Interactions

The Energy Restoration Protocol emphasizes plant based Raw Foods, some of which contain compounds that may interact with medications:

- Vitamin K in leafy greens may affect blood thinners (warfarin).

- Potassium-rich foods may interact with certain blood pressure or heart medications.
- Calcium-rich foods may affect absorption of some medications.
- High fiber may affect absorption of some medications.

These interactions are generally manageable with medical oversight and are not reasons to avoid the protocol. However, your health care provider should know about significant dietary changes so they can monitor for interactions.

Inform your health care provider of significant dietary changes and monitor for any medication interactions.

INDIVIDUAL VARIATION AND PERSONALIZATION

Results vary significantly based on individual circumstances.

The case studies in this manifesto represent successful implementations, but not everyone will experience the same results or timeline. Individual variation is influenced by:

- Genetics and genetic predisposition
- Age and life stage
- Medical history and existing conditions
- Current medications
- Severity of existing disease
- Degree of metabolic dysfunction
- Adherence to protocol
- Activity level and exercise
- Stress levels and sleep quality
- Social support and family dynamics
- Environmental factors
- Starting point (disease prevention vs. disease reversal)

Your results may differ significantly from case studies presented. This does not mean the protocol is ineffective for you; it means individual circumstances vary.

WHEN TO SEEK EMERGENCY MEDICAL CARE

Seek immediate emergency medical care if you experience:

- Chest pain or pressure
- Severe shortness of breath
- Severe abdominal pain
- Severe dizziness or fainting
- Severe headache with confusion or vision changes
- Signs of stroke (facial drooping, arm weakness, speech difficulty)

- Severe allergic reaction
- Blood sugar levels dangerously high or low (if diabetic)
- Severe psychiatric symptoms or suicidal thoughts
- Severe bleeding or hemorrhage
- Any other life-threatening emergency symptoms

Do not delay seeking emergency care to try protocol interventions.

FOOD ALLERGIES AND INTOLERANCES

Carefully assess for food allergies and intolerances before implementation.

The Energy Restoration Protocol emphasizes whole plant foods. For most people, these foods are safe and nutritious. However, some individuals have allergies or intolerances to:

- Nuts and seeds (potentially severe allergies)
- Legumes (beans, lentils, peanuts some people have intolerances)
- Grains (gluten sensitivity, celiac disease)
- Specific vegetables or fruits
- Soy (present in some plant-based products)

Know your allergies and intolerances before implementing. Modify the protocol to avoid foods you're allergic or intolerant to. Chapter 17 provides guidance for implementing the protocol with common allergies.

If you develop new allergic reactions during implementation, discontinue the suspected food and consult your health care provider.

NUTRIENT DEFICIENCY RISKS

Plant-based diets require attention to certain nutrients:

- Vitamin B12: Not naturally abundant in plant foods. Supplementation or fortified foods are essential.
- Vitamin D: Limited plant sources. Sun exposure, fortified foods, or supplementation may be needed.
- Iron: Plant-based (non-heme) iron is less bioavailable than animal iron. Adequate intake requires attention to sources and absorption enhancement.
- Calcium: Adequate plant sources exist, but intake must be intentional.
- Omega-3 fatty acids: Plant sources provide ALA; conversion to DHA/EPA is limited. Supplementation may be appropriate.
- Zinc: Plant-based sources are available but require attention.

If you have concerns about specific nutrient deficiencies, work with a registered dietitian or health care provider.

EXERCISE AND PHYSICAL ACTIVITY CONSIDERATIONS

Exercise recommendations assume reasonable baseline health.

Chapter 18 provides movement and exercise guidance for various populations. However:

- Individuals with cardiovascular conditions should consult their cardiologist before starting exercise programs.
- Individuals with joint problems should consult physical therapists about movement.
- Individuals with balance problems should focus on safe, supported movement.
- Individuals with chronic pain should work with health care providers on appropriate movement.
- Severe deconditioning requires gradual, medically supervised exercise progression.

Consult your health care provider before starting new exercise programs if you have any health conditions or concerns.

REALISTIC EXPECTATIONS

Understand realistic timelines and outcomes:

- Timeline: Health improvements occur gradually. Dramatic improvements often appear within 1–3 months, but complete reversal of long-standing disease may take 6+ months.
- Incomplete reversal: Not all disease markers normalize completely. Some chronic conditions may improve substantially but not fully resolve.
- Medication dependence: Some people with certain conditions may require ongoing medications even after substantial improvement.
- Individual ceiling: Your best health may be different from others'. This does not mean the protocol failed.
- Maintenance required: Benefits require ongoing protocol adherence. Returning to processed foods typically results in return of disease.
- Genetic ceiling: Genetics play a role. Optimal health via the protocol may look different for different people.

Have realistic expectations and celebrate improvements rather than expecting perfect outcomes.

RESPONSIBILITY AND LIABILITY

By reading and implementing anything in this manifesto, you acknowledge:

1. You have consulted with your health care provider about implementing these changes (or chose not to, taking full responsibility).

2. You understand this is not medical advice.
3. You understand individual results vary.
4. You are responsible for your own health decisions and outcomes.
5. You will monitor your health and seek medical care if needed.
6. You understand medications may need adjustment under medical supervision.
7. You will not blame the author for outcomes resulting from your implementation.

The author accepts no liability for health outcomes resulting from implementation of the Energy Restoration Protocol. While the protocol has supported health transformation for many people, the author cannot be held responsible for individual health outcomes, medication interactions, adverse events, or any consequences resulting from your implementation choices.

WORKING WITH YOUR HEALTH CARE PROVIDER

Recommended approach:

1. Share this manifesto with your health care provider.
2. Discuss the Energy Restoration Protocol with your provider.
3. Get explicit permission and guidance before implementing.
4. Be transparent about any changes you make.
5. Have regular medical appointments and blood work.
6. Report any concerns or adverse effects to your provider.
7. Work together on medication adjustments if needed.
8. Use your provider as a resource and partner.

Most health care providers appreciate patients who are engaged with their health and open to lifestyle changes. Open communication is key.

Final Note

This manifesto is offered in service.

The author believes deeply that the Energy Restoration Protocol represents a genuine pathway to health transformation. This manifesto represents years of work to share this understanding clearly and comprehensively.

However, the author also understands that health care is personal, individual, and complex. There is no single approach that works for everyone. Your health care provider, knowing your full medical history and individual circumstances, is the appropriate guide for your personal health decisions.

Use this manifesto as a resource. Work with your health care team. Take responsibility for your own health. And trust that when you align with nature and provide your body what it actually needs, profound healing becomes possible.

Summary: What to Do Before You Start

- o   1. Read this entire disclaimer
- o   2. Consult with your health care provider
- o   3. Discuss the Energy Restoration Protocol with your provider
- o   4. Get explicit medical clearance if you have health conditions or take medications
- o   5. Understand realistic expectations
- o   6. Commit to transparency with your health care team
- o   7. Begin implementation with medical support and oversight
- o   8. Monitor your health and report changes to your provider
- o   9. Be patient with the process
- o   10. Celebrate improvements

IN NATURE WE TRUST. Work *with* nature. Work *with* your medical team. Work *with* your body.

Your health journey is personal. Make it informed. Make it safe. Make it yours.

A PERSONAL REQUEST
FROM AXAY SHAH

Your Feedback Matters

You've finished reading this manifesto. You now understand the Energy Restoration Protocol. You understand that disease is not inevitable. You understand that you have power over your health.

But this book is not the end. It's the beginning.

The real work happens in your life in your kitchen, in your daily choices, in your transformation. And I want to hear about it.

Your feedback, your questions, your transformation stories, these matter deeply. They're not just reviews. They're proof of possibility for others who are considering this path.

How to Share Your Feedback

Whether you purchased this book through Amazon, Google Play Books, Apple Books, received it as a gift, borrowed it from a library, found it at a local bookstore, or discovered it online your feedback matters. Here are the two best ways to share your experience:

ON AMAZON

If you purchased this book through Amazon, a review there is incredibly valuable. Share:

- What resonated with you
- How you're implementing the protocol
- Changes you've noticed
- Questions or suggestions

Amazon reviews help others discover this work. Your honest feedback, positive or constructive, guides readers and builds community.

ON INNATUREWETRUST.NET

Visit *innaturewetrust.net* and share your experience:

- Your health transformation
- Obstacles you overcame
- Questions about implementation
- Testimonial about the book's impact

This is your dedicated space to connect with other readers and share your journey.

VIA EMAIL

hello@InNatureWeTrust.net

Contact directly with your story, questions, or feedback. Share what's working. Share what's challenging. This helps me refine and improve guidance for others following this path.

SHARE THIS BOOK WITH OTHERS

This manifesto exists to serve people who are ready for transformation. If you know people who:

- Struggle with chronic disease and want to understand why
- Are interested in disease prevention and optimal health
- Want to understand the connection between food and health
- Are curious about plant-based nutrition
- Are seeking a unified framework for understanding health
- Are ready to take responsibility for their own health

Share This Book with Them

This is not about sales. This is about possibility. When you share this manifesto, you're saying, "I believe your health can be different. I believe transformation is possible. I believe this book can show you how."

You become a messenger of possibility for others.

How to Share

Easy ways to share:

- Recommend on social media (tag RawFoodiest.com, mention InNatureWeTrust.net)
- Gift the book to someone you care about
- Recommend in health/wellness groups

- Share your transformation story and mention how this book helped
- Leave a review and encourage others to read it
- Discuss specific chapters with interested friends

Building Community

The most powerful transformations happen in the community. When you share this work, you're not just recommending a book. You're building a community of people aligned with:

- Trusting nature
- Taking responsibility for health
- Understanding energy as the foundation
- Creating optimal health through daily choices
- Supporting each other in transformation

This community is your community, becomes stronger as more people discover this framework and implement it.

Your Transformation Inspires Others

Never underestimate the power of your own transformation. When people see you:

- With abundant energy at an age when decline is "normal"
- Free from medications that seemed inevitable
- Sleeping well, thinking clearly, emotionally stable
- Athletic and vital and thriving

They think, "If they can do it, maybe I can too."

Your transformation is permission for others. Your feedback and your sharing become proof of possibility.

The Ripple Effect

This is how real change happens. Not top-down from institutions or corporations. But person-to-person. One person transforms, shares that transformation, helps someone else transform, who then helps others.

Ripples expanding outward. One person at a time. One transformation at a time.

You hold that power. Your feedback. Your sharing. Your willingness to tell others: "This book changed how I understand my health."

Thank You

Thank you for reading this manifesto. Thank you for engaging with this framework. Thank you for considering that your health is your responsibility and your creation.

Whether you implement the protocol fully, partially, or simply use pieces of it you are already moving toward better alignment with nature and with your own body.

If you share this work with others, you multiply that impact.

Three Simple Asks

1. **Leave feedback** On Amazon, InNatureWeTrust.net, or via email. Share your honest response to this manifesto.
2. **Share your journey** If you implement the protocol, I'd love to hear about your experience. Your story helps others.
3. **Recommend to others** Share this book with people you care about who are ready for transformation. Be a messenger of possibility.

Stay Connected

- **INNATUREWETRUST.net** Book home, feedback, resources
- **axayshah.com** Author platform, all projects
- **Raw Foodiest** Coaching programs, community, webinars
- **Social media** Share your journey, tag #InNatureWeTrust

Final Words

"If it's not made by Mother Nature, it's not going on my plate."

Your health. Your responsibility. Your power. Your choice.
IN NATURE WE TRUST.
Life is Energy and Energy is Life.
With gratitude and in service,

—AXAY SHAH

Author, IN NATURE WE TRUST: *Health Manifesto*

Founder, RAWFOODIEST.COM

Sixty-Six-Year-Young Marathon Runner

Twenty-One Years Documented Health Transformation

Please share this work. Help build a world where health is understood, disease is prevented, and transformation is possible.
IN NATURE WE TRUST

THIRTY-DAY WORKSHEET:
TRACK YOUR TRANSFORMATION

Your journey to optimal health begins with awareness. The Thirty-Day Worksheet is your personal tracking tool to monitor your progress as you implement the Energy Restoration Protocol.

Why Use the Worksheet?

Tracking isn't just about numbers. It's about awareness. As you document your daily choices—the foods you eat, your energy levels, your sleep quality, your mood, your physical performance—you'll begin to see patterns. You'll notice what works. You'll feel the connection between your choices and your results.

This is powerful. This is motivating. This is how transformation becomes real.

What You'll Track:

- Daily food choices and energy levels
- Sleep quality and duration
- Physical activity and movement
- Mental clarity and mood
- Specific health markers (blood pressure, weight, energy, digestion)
- Obstacles and victories
- How you feel, day by day

MAKE IT FUN

This isn't clinical. This is your personal health story. Celebrate small wins. Notice improvements you didn't expect. Share your progress with your Raw Foodiest community.

DOWNLOAD YOUR THIRTY-DAY WORKSHEET

Visit: *https://rawfoodiest.com/complete-program-guide/* or scan the QR code to access your worksheet instantly..

Your transformation starts with one day. Then another. Then thirty. Let the worksheet be your guide.

ABOUT THE AUTHOR

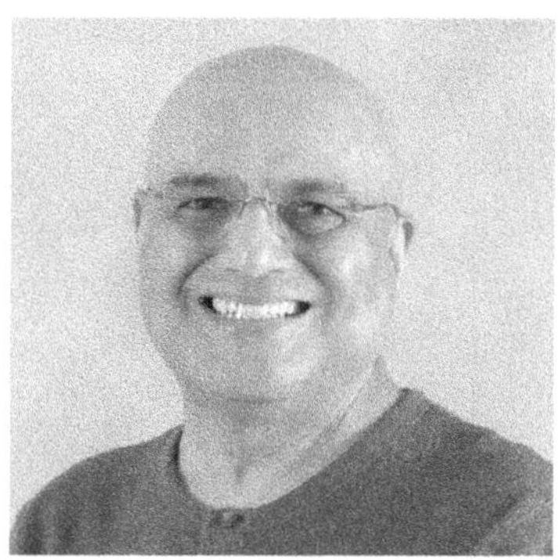

Axay Shah is a raw food educator and author who has spent over sixteen years documenting what becomes possible when you align with nature.

At fifty, diagnosed with Type 2 prediabetes, he approached it differently. Rather than accept a disease trajectory, he became curious. What if he experimented with aligning his nutrition with nature? Today, at sixty-six years young, he stands as living proof: sixteen years of documented reversal without medications, eight completed marathons, and health markers that exceed most people half his age all from a simple decision to experiment.

Born in Kolkata, raised in Mumbai, and based in Los Angeles since 1985, Axay brings a cross-cultural perspective to wellness. Through RawFoodiest.com, he has built a thriving community of health-seeking people, creating blog posts and YouTube videos focused on education over prescription.

Beyond his work as an educator, Axay is a poet (pen name: Bachu), karaoke singer, drummer, marathon runner, beekeeper, gardener, and pond keeper. He lives his philosophy daily: "Life is Beautiful. Good health is the foundation. Everything else follows."

He remains a humble seeker, learning something new every day, inviting open-minded health seekers to discover what becomes possible when energy is genuinely restored.

This manifesto is his sixteen-year testimony.

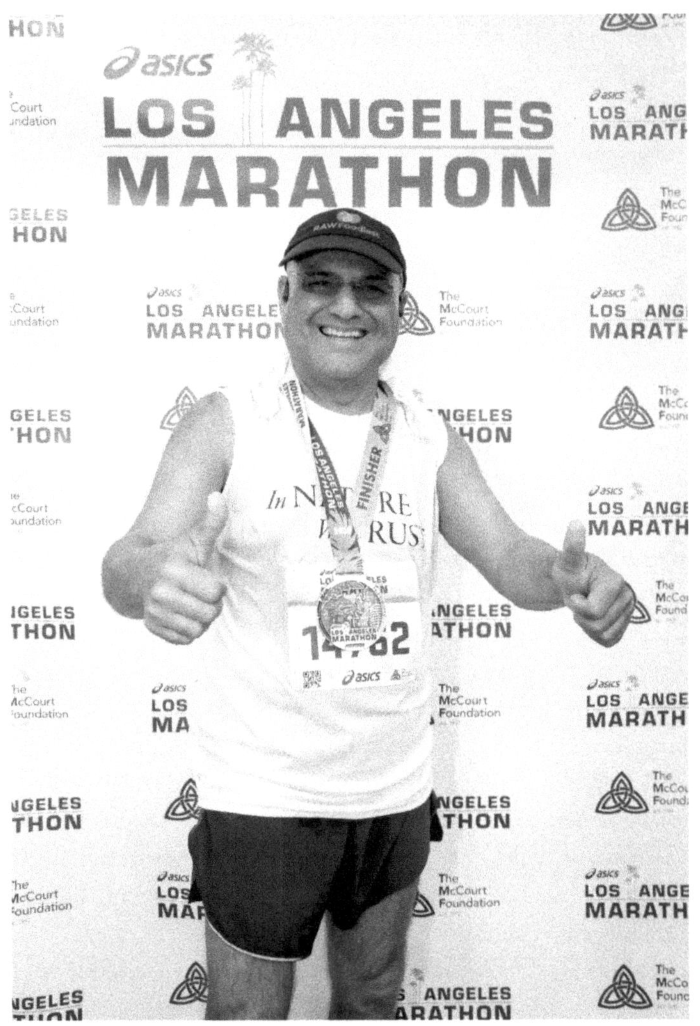

I crossed the finish line of my eighth marathon on March 8th, 2026.